Indian Superfoods

Reader Reviews on the Juggernaut App

'Rujuta, you are a revolution…the Rujuta Revolution… thank u once again for giving a new life to our dying traditions and foods and most importantly our Super Grandmoms'—**Priyanka Jha**

'I have always admired your work and this book is no exception. Thank you for enlightening us with this everlasting Indian food wisdom. We truly are a country of what they call "Superfoods". Perhaps it's good to have a sweet tooth 😬'—**Meghana Badal**

'Hats off to you Rujuta….very well informative book every youngsters should read…so much information…given in detail. I have read all your books and all are in my shelf. I am following your diet for the past five years. I am always energetic, active and I never starve and have strength to look after my granddaughter. Thank you for writing such a wonderful book…You keep on writing…and I will go on adding it on my shelf…and also pass on to people who need it. Thank you once again. Love you'—**Desai**

'Very informative and desi! I felt like dancing after reading positive about my favorite aliv ladu 😀 like all other books by Rujuta, this one is interesting and offers a wow moment after every chapter. TOI, please do not publish reports with snaps of goras having lunch with farmers that have found instant money in growing quinoa...instead, print a chapter from this book to celebrate Indian superfoods and advertise these foods to help ecological and economic growth. Thank you Rujuta, to revive and help sustain this knowledge that was on its way to be forgotten. as with her other books, I'm going to gift this one to my near and dear ones. Thanks Chiki for making the book so affordable 👍'—Uma Kulkarni

'This is an eye–opener book really. Coming from a reputed nutritionist the book demolishes many myths of the food front and gives respect to old age wisdom of grandmom. What has been said is logical and juxtaposed with relevant studies. We need to read more things like this to save health and save environment too'—Jitendra

'Apart from you and a couple of famous YouTube fitness guys from US, no one explains rice better!!! Thank you for getting me out of my misery. I don't have to eat brown rice now and be constipated. I can eat my very own varan bhaat, macchi bhaat daal!'—Aditya Tawde

'I have always been a fan of Rujuta Diwekar's books right from her first book that I had read. Her approach towards a diet has always impressed me and whoever I suggest her books to. Her books are for keeping. Her books are guidebooks for a healthy life. Thanks Rujuta for explaining the super foods of India'—Sanjiv T. Badgujar

'I am a big fan of Rujuta and try to follow her way of eating local traditional food as much as possible. After reading this book, I am looking at sugar and cashew with a new perspective. Due to her previous books I started eating my fav ghee religiously and I can clearly see the difference in my skin and also get compliments for my clear and glowing skin. Thank you Rujuta for bringing my fav ambadi chi bhaji back on the table. lovvv you'—**Rupali**

'I have always loved Rujuta's books. And this one ladies and gentlemen...is certainly going to go on my most recommended list. BRILLIANT!'—**Rashmi Praveen**

'I have found nirvana after reading this book. I always thought how we could fear food so much and that too native ones passed on through centuries. This book has thrashed all that is irrelevant and fearful. Thanks Rujuta... will forever be indebted to u. I can't stop sharing this one with my near and dear ones...off to happy wholesome eating now'—**Sunil Gaikwad**

'Awesome to the core...her simple, funny and fresh style makes us learned, happy and enthusiastic respectively. Eager to eat all these foods over and over again with a better understanding of their nutrient content...luckily, i never stopped eating them earlier! A hamper containing these 10 (or at least the dry 5) superfoods is a good gift at events, parties, birthdays! Thanks a lot, Rujuta, u make local delicacies look totally nutritive and fashionable to consume! They are, in their all glory!'—**Suruchi Bapat**

'Perfect! This is the kind of myth busting we require today. Hats off!!'—**Noopur**

'It's simply awesome. You explained us how the food which we avoid daily are actually SUPERFOODS. Our dadi, nani, mom, masi always told us to eat these superfoods but we avoided it because they never gave us the satisfactory answer of our question 'why' but now there is no reason to avoid. Thanks a ton. Rujuta, u r a revolution. Wish I could meet u someday'—**Ankur Gupta**

'Very informative, useful, clear many doubts...nice experience to read...waiting for new book on other superfood... or other topics'—**Falguni Gandhi**

'Thanks, Rujuta. Now I realise I have been so wrong and must say rude to my mother who has been telling me for ages all the good things she has learnt. And me a spoilt brat would correct her for not being updated about the current trend in superfoods. Going back home to spend some time with her now'—**Dhanashree Tabib**

'OMG...everything that we had been told over the years and still took for granted is proven and scientifically explained. A must–read for all who are proud of our culture and ancient wisdom'—**Meghna**

Indian Superfoods

Rujuta Diwekar

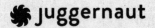

JUGGERNAUT BOOKS

KS House, 118 Shahpur Jat, New Delhi 110049, India

First published by Juggernaut Books 2016

10 9

ISBN 9788193237236

Typeset in Adobe Caslon Pro by R. Ajith Kumar, New Delhi

Printed at Manipal Technologies Limited

Contents

Introduction   1

Ghee: The Fat Burner   21

Kokum: The Natural Antacid   43

Banana: The Recharger   57

Kaju: The Antidepressant   71

Ambadi: The Stomach-Soother   85

Rice: The Grain That Sustains   97

Coconut: The Calmer   109

Aliv: The Beauty Pill   121

Jackfruit: The Fertility Booster   131

Sugar: The Anti-Ageing Secret   145

Appendix: Regional Names of Aliv, Ambadi   175
and Kokum

A Note on the Author   177

Contents

Introduction

1

2

3

4

5

6

Appendix

Notes

Introduction

'If you want to be a super hit, you must find young women to follow you,' said a casting director to an aspiring actor at a coffee shop in Oshiwara. A friend from Italy who's also a famous DJ asked me over chai and toast, early one morning, 'Who do you think made the Beatles?' I drew a blank and raised my eyebrows. 'Teenage women,' she announced. 'You get the women to follow you, the rest of the world follows.' I thought of my time in Masai Mara, when a lioness walked away without giving a damn and the lion immediately got up and followed her. 'See that,' whispered my guide. 'Always male follow female, always. That's the rule.'

Once upon a time, not very long ago, it was

the women in our homes who controlled what, when and how much we ate. And both the genders participated in food decisions and preparations. Till that time there was no such thing as diabesity. The latest buzzword, diabesity is the burden of obesity and diabetes that the rich of the developing world carry. That's you and me, rich enough for phones, Wi-Fi and 4G.

This richness/technology has shifted the decision of what to eat, how much to eat and when to eat away from women. This power now rests with nameless, faceless pages which download at a crazy speed and inform us about the latest weight-loss aid. Who ate what and knocked off how much is now helping us decide what and how much to eat. None of these pages know anything about our lives, our likes or our wives but they tell us what to eat. They promise us weight loss with just eating something, this something always has to be bought, and it's always expensive, unpronounceable and strikes us as a revolutionary idea. It's also stuff that your grandma doesn't recognize as food, doesn't grow locally and is invariably tasteless. It makes you feel that if you somehow suffer your way through it, then surely at the end of it there will be that all-elusive weight loss.

Is There an Indian Superfood?

Statistics though prove that less than 20 per cent people are successful in keeping the weight off after they have lost it. Not just numbers but your experience will tell you that it's easy to knock the weight off but tough to keep it off. It seems to find a way back to your body, climbs into places where fat never existed and this time stays like it means to stay forever. Nothing, however crash, latest or expensive seems to knock it off.

Into this mix comes the superfood – a food item that promises a miracle and comes from somewhere exotic. Acacia seeds, goji berries, kale – the world seems to discover a superfood every week. There's so much talk about them in the press that the word itself seems to have no meaning. What's a superfood then really, do they even exist, asked my editor, Chiki.

Is it something that has more nutrition than others? Is it more powerful?

For me superfoods are foods that, like true love, have stood the test of time. They have at least these five things in common:

1. They grow naturally in the same land you live
2. They are rich in micronutrients and taste
3. Every part of the crop/plant can be used in unique ways
4. They encourage diversity in your diet
5. They lead to a sustainable lifestyle, help local economy and make sound ecological sense

Superfoods Are Always Local

I recently attended a course called the 'Future of Food' in Potsdam, Germany, and there we were, participants from all across the developing world, learning about what it would take to feed the world in 2050 – with an exploding population of 9 billion people and the climate change, we are in a lot of trouble. And the focus constantly came back to this – **Future foods are local foods – and people in the**

developing world give up eating the local foods because it's less prestigious to eat them. And these local superfoods, which in ancient times and not so ancient times (like sixty years ago) were celebrated for their therapeutic, weight-loss and well-being properties, are now undervalued or simply lost. Then the West adopts them as 'novel foods' for weight loss and well-being and they get a second lease of life.

So curcumin enters the health store as an antidote to fatigue and obesity but we don't even know that it's haldi. The moringa powder that we mix in water for omega 3 and stamina is just the drumstick in the sambar and that amaranth is simply the rajgeera chikki you get at railway stations. While everyone in India knows how much dal to add to rice to make khichdi, someone in the West is studying its proportions to earn a PhD. And they will probably also pursue a post-doc in how the proportions change when the person is sick or when seasons change or whether you want to turn it into a dosa or an idli. We take food wisdom so much for granted that we don't even recognize it as something of great importance.

If nothing, at least let us acknowledge that we are copying the food habits of people who are copying us, or our grandmothers more specifically. So we are just dheela copycats. The stuff worth copying is not jumping queues, five-day workweeks, respecting pedestrian rights, etc., but we are not interested in that.

Sukhasana

It's not just food but even habits that need to be local. Sukhasana (easy pose or happy pose) is nothing but the cross-legged posture that you assume while sitting on the floor to eat. You can start with at least one meal a week in the sukhasana posture and then allow it to grow organically into your life. You will notice that meals in the sukhasana posture always feel lighter, tastier and even happier.

Stanford University researchers have recently built the squatty potty, one that replicates the

Asian pot, and already sold more than a million of them. They are not too far away from coming up with research to prove that eating meals on the floor in a cross-legged posture is better for the colon, blood–brain barrier and what have you. So you can either do it now as a practise of the culture you are born into or you can do it later, once someone acquires a patent on it.

Superfoods Are All about Food Traditions

Superfoods are compassionate and wise, like the Buddhist deities Avalokiteshwara and Manjushri, because without them in equal measure, there is no real power. At least according to the lama in Tabo monastery in Spiti, and I believe him.

Superfoods don't just stand the test of time but they are compassionate to the other plants that grow around them. They coexist, striking a symbiotic relationship with the soil, climate and living beings on their land. They are versatile, like Asha Bhosle, who can sing the bhajan and cabaret like she means it.

Superfoods can be used as therapy, will lend themselves to rituals and even bring income to those who grow them. In that sense these are the wise foods, ones that know they must bring pleasure to the palate, nourishment to the body and even work as medicine when required.

And it's exactly this quality of our native grains, fruits and vegetables that gives them the power to be used in every possible form. In that sense they are not just powerful but also empowering foods. The bark and stems, the raw and the ripe fruit, the leaves and the seeds, every part is usable, unique in its therapeutic properties, and nourishment value and tasty to boot.

While one part can be turned into a sabzi, another part will provide edible oil and all this while retaining nitrogen (natural fertilizer) in the soil, beautifying the locale and providing shade to those who wish to sit next to it. Basically, indigenous crops do what big food companies don't – they own their waste. They are in fact zero-waste – from being used as a natural fertilizer to being turned into a jhadoo or even into a fabric, they leave behind zero footprint. They are ecologically smart.

Double Burden of Malnourishment

The world is facing a double burden of malnourishment. Where the poor are denied the easy-to-assimilate protein that comes from dal–chawal, for example, and this leads to deformities or even death. And the rich, because of their disconnect with reality, don't think of dal–chawal or khichdi as protein and want to eat more meat for protein or simply eat quinoa salad. And this switch from local to more industrialized or exotic food is at the root of diabesity. Today, the cost of obesity is 2.1 trillion dollars – that's as high as armed conflicts. So every time you tsk tsk about terrorism around the globe, know that this culture of eating certain things to receive a certain nutrient which magically turns us thinner is, at least in terms of expenditure, the same as armed conflict.

National Geographic brought into focus five steps that would help create a more sustainable environment and reduce this double burden of malnourishment on the globe. These are:

1. Freeze agricultural footprint (eat regional)
2. Grow more on the same land (rotate crops)
3. Use resources more efficiently (optimize water usage)
4. Shift diets (diversify) (eat less meat)
5. Reduce waste

Superfoods Are Often Forgotten

Some of the superfoods in this book you may have known, some are unknown or less known, while some have been celebrated since the time of the Vedas.

Based on popular perception, you can divide them into these three groups:

1. So yummy that they can't possibly be healthy – ghee, rice, coconut, banana
2. Too local or desi to have any fat-burning or other health benefits – jackfruit, sugar cane, kaju
3. Never heard of them – aliv, kokum, ambadi

Or we can have another type of division:

1. Full of cholesterol – ghee, coconut, kaju
2. Too sweet or too many calories – rice, jackfruit, sugar cane, banana
3. Too low profile to be useful – aliv, kokum, ambadi

Now, of course, as you read on, you will see how these perceptions are totally wrong. But what you should know right away is that these superfoods are not just your pill to weight loss but to an irreversible and sustainable weight loss. And besides weight loss these will make you look good – right now, with glowing skin, lustrous hair and flat stomach, and after you are gone as responsible citizens who didn't kill the earth and economy in their greed to get thin. And while looking good, it gives you the other benefits of good looks – of sustainable blood sugars, of a thriving libido and fertility levels and of a calm state of mind. After all, a skinny waist is wasted without good sex, stable sugars and sharp intellect.

The Return of the Langot

There's no such thing as an original idea, Rujuta, said my seventy-five-year-old wise man, there's only original execution. He was bang on target. Take the case of nappies. All of us in the developing countries, the rich specifically, have switched to these plastic and foam filled nappies as a cool, hassle-free and smart alternative to the langot. The latest trend among the super-rich, cool and eco-conscious of New York, however, is the langot, as the mass-produced nappies give

---

rashes to babies and create ecological waste. The weekly stock for the 'cloth diapers' arrives at your home, and at the end of the week it gets collected, washed and dried using hot water and plant-based detergents. If you tell this to your grandma she's gonna have an ROFL moment. You and she could have a similar business idea. You do the website, she puts in the intellectual capital, you two have a roaring success of a business and it's good for babies and the earth.

Superfoods Always Work with Others

The most endearing thing about these superfoods is that they are not vain – you have to eat them with other things for them to work. They coexist, not just with each other but even among themselves. Rice, for example, has hundreds of indigenous varieties just in Odisha – there's a sticky rice for the lactating mother and another one for the young groom that he must have the night before his wedding to please his wife. The banana also has multiple varieties, so do sugar cane and coconut, each one of them. The same goes for our others. So they are not here to stake claim to be the only ten foods that you must eat but simply to say that these ten foods you must eat along with the other local stuff.

After all, these ten superfoods are smart, they know that diversity is the key to survival and sustainability. Rice wants to go with dal and a blob of ghee. The ghee wants to be on your bhakri, roti and even on your feet. The kaju will go with rava or moong to turn into a halwa or with jaggery to become a chikki. The jackfruit will lend itself beautifully to your biryani or become your midday snack. The banana can be rolled inside a roti for lunch or you can mix it with other veggies for undhiyo. The kokum likes the company of sprouts or even chaat. The ambadi will add more bite to your millets, while the aliv is happy to blend into sugar or jaggery with coconut or simply to garnish your sandwich.

As you will see in the following chapters, it's the combination of foods that performs magic in our bodies. Superfoods are also great at enabling other foods and nutrients to perform their miracles.

You Have to Style Your Own Superfood

Endless possibilities is a super thing. **And the body after all is used to a wholesome and not an isolation approach.** So when you read about these foods, don't start eating them in bulk quantities or with just hot water first thing in the morning. In all the chapters I have listed how to eat these foods, but the best way to eat them is through your regional food culture and using your home recipes. Call your mom and ask her how to make or use the foods that you read about. Or better still, have a family get-together where you document how the food is prepared, served and stored with inputs from the grandparents, aunts and uncles. Make a family heritage piece of all the foods that you eat in your own unique style, or frame a recipe and give it as gift or hang it on your wall. Who knows, forty years on, your family can sell these for millions, like an art piece that not only appreciates in value but till then gives you sukoon, and good health too.

How Much to Eat

Staying silent while eating is the most undervalued aspect of good nutrition. Don't talk, don't read, don't surf, just eat. It will actually put you in touch with yourself and then you will hear the voice of your stomach. Your stomach will guide you in eating the right quantities at every meal. It will slow down the pace at which you are consuming. It will make you feel lighter, younger, calmer with every bite. The space will reverberate with inner peace and you will hear a voice in your head go:

Pakakarta tatha bhokta, annadata sukhi bhava.

May the person who cooks, the one who eats and the one who provides the food, may all be happy. And just like that, peace will return to the world, at least to your world.

In summary, superfood is food that moves beyond just health and nutrition. It suits your genetic make-up, it blends into not just your regional cuisine, but even into your culture. It tells you a story, of the history of your land, its flavour reminds you of the good laughs you shared with your cousins, its aroma makes you feel like your grandma is still in the room, watching over you, giggling with you, urging you to eat just one more bite.

1

Ghee
The Fat Burner

'*Yatha jeevet, sukham jeevet, runam krutva, ghrutam pibet.*' For as long as you live, live happily, and even if you have to take a loan, ensure that you can drink ghee. In India's 'panchamrit', the five nectars of life, milk and milk products dominate – and of these ghee is the king. But then we are getting maha dairy averse these days and are wanting to fix the blame for our paunches on poor lactose but that's only when we are not blaming gluten for it. 'Keep that sarcasm in check,' I hear my partner's voice in my head. So I will, and will tell you another story, the short story of casteism in our country.

For a country that is still trying to break free from the shackles of the caste system, here's what the wise have said – *Jeshthatwam janmana naiv, gunaiihi jeshthatwam uchyate, gunat gurutwam aayati, dugdham, dadhim, ghrutam kramat.'* Being born into a certain family doesn't make you better than others, it's your virtues that set you apart; milk, curd and ghee, all come from the cow but the one with the highest status is ghee and that is because it makes the greatest contribution to the well-being of our body, mind and soul.

From birth to death, like the grain of rice, ghee is an inherent part of your life. If you are Hindu, your body, and mine, will receive some ghee before it gets burned – the only choice we have is wood or electric, ghee is non-negotiable. Check this out the next time you are at a funeral.

The Super-Fat

It's not just what our forefathers said, ghee is *the* super-fat. What makes it so special? Four little letters that spell a miracle – SCFA – short chain fatty acids, which are the world's top-performing fats. Alongside the usual functions of fat, they promote fat burning from stubborn fat areas of the body, healthy bacteria in the gut, the health of your heart and even buddhi, the brain's ability to discriminate. But isn't ghee super unhealthy? The fat that we should be using as little as possible?

If buddhi worked, you would be able to ask yourself (because arguments with others are a waste of time and you waste your time when you don't question yourself) – why is it that I eat a Marie biscuit without fear of a heart attack and avoid ghee on my dal–bhaat or roti out of fear of a heart attack?

Why do I accept the long chain fatty acids in the biscuits that can oxidize my tissues, accelerate my ageing and ruin my nutrient to calorie ratio with ease? Is it because they are low cal or because my dietician/doctor approved of it? Why did I ignore what my dadi told me – *Beta, ghee khao*. Did she care less about me than my doctor who had to look in my chart to know my name?

Hasn't dadi's wisdom stood the test of time unlike medical advice which changes its messages every year? After all, didn't the USFDA admit in 2015 that there is no reason to avoid fat in one's diet and that there's no link between cholesterol and heart disease – something they had strongly maintained since the 1970s. So I gave up on ghee, coconut, groundnuts and cashews, all local and all recommended by dadi, out of fear of a heart attack because they have cholesterol – only to be proved wrong.

Food knowledge flows like an unbroken stream from generation to generation till it's broken down by someone who is unrelated to us telling us what to eat and how to look. We have a storehouse of wisdom at home who only gives out food messages that have stood the test of time through observations on real humans in real-life conditions. Instead, we opt to live by research on mice or some tiny population that's not even genetically similar to us, who have been studied for much shorter than even a lifetime and where every discrepancy is eliminated and conditions standardized.

Traditional food wisdom	Modern medical advice on food
Has stood the test of time for centuries	Changes every few years
Has real humans in free living conditions as subjects	Has mice or small sample set of humans in controlled conditions as subjects
Accounts for all variations in climate, season, genetic eating behaviour, etc.	Eliminates all discrepancies

And this flawed research is spinning off an entire food industry, for example, of oils with hearts on the packaging. As it happens, most of these vegetable oils have now been proven to be unhealthy. And then as I shifted to other oils for the omega 3, after all I know myself to be a man of reason and research, did I notice that NICE (the UK health guidelines) officially removed omega 3 as a nutrient that helps heart health way back in June 2014? Did the people who asked me to switch to olive oil for heart health update me on this? Or maybe I didn't care. Is it too far-fetched to believe that my grandma got it right? Eat ghee and eat it as much as you like.

The GI Joe

The addition of ghee to your meals reduces the glycaemic index of food. Now I know you went off ghee the minute you were declared diabetic but this is based on reduction of calories without giving a damn about where these calories come from and how they affect your blood sugar levels. PCOD, diabetes and obesity arise out of insulin-resistance and one way of improving this is to eat meals that have a low glycaemic index.

The reason why there are such combos as dal–chawal–ghee, roti–shakkar–ghee, puran-poli–ghee, modak–ghee, etc., in our culture is that ghee reduces the glycaemic index of these meals. The addition of any fat to food reduces its glycaemic index and ghee is brilliant in this regard. The magic of ghee isn't just that it's the world's most high-functioning fat. It's also that it's a wonderful partner to other foods, complementing them to work better and harder for us.

So ghee regulates blood sugars and that reduces the risk of developing metabolic syndrome. This ensures that there is a slow, steady rise in blood sugars and better energy levels through the day. Feel that afternoon slump? Add ghee to your lunch. Ghee won't just help combat diabetes and obesity but it will prevent heart diseases too. And if you are already affected by these conditions, then know that ghee will still come to your rescue.

Deep-frying in ghee also comes from the same wisdom. Making Shankar pala, suhali, mathri or even luchis that use fibre-less maida? How do I enjoy these delicacies without disturbing my blood sugars? Simply deep-fry them and in the best available fatty acid – ghee. The slow, steady climb in the blood sugars also makes it easy for the body to effectively assimilate the herbs and spices that these meals contain. Also, as a cooking medium, ghee has among the highest smoke points (measure of how quickly a fat oxidizes, or goes bad, when heated).

Do you know that every time you bake or use any other method of robbing your meal of essential fats like ghee, the glycemic index of your meal stays high? That means faster ageing and predisposition to metabolic syndrome. So much for the air fryer.

The Ghee, Pregnancy and Vitamin D Connection

Every pregnant woman was traditionally given tons of ghee right from the first period she missed to the period she got post-pregnancy and all was well in the world then. Not many women developed hypothyroidism just because they had delivered a baby. They had the support of the most unique fatty acid made in the sophisticated lab of their own mommies – the kitchen. And then this SCFA helped them get pregnant, keep calm during pregnancy, deliver smoothly and lose all the weight at the delivery table. Now I can give you some solid thermodynamic principles about how this happens and sound very intelligent, but since I am not, I will just tell you some school-level biology and what we studied about fat-soluble vitamins.

So thyroid is a gland that has to work overtime during pregnancy because it's your T3 (one of the thyroid hormones) that takes active part and supports the optimum growth of the fetus. Lactation is another kind of biological burden that your thyroid has to bear. If you cut down ghee because it is full of calories or other such BS, then you are not getting this magical SCFA, and because vitamin D is a fat-soluble vitamin, you are not assimilating enough of that either. Now not just your pregnancy, your diet or lack of a good diet is putting an additional burden on the thyroid, because vitamin D plays a critical role in regulating the thyroid glands. You have made a choice to get pregnant but the choice of not eating ghee is coming out of the fear of getting fat. And fear only comes out of avidya, the opposite of knowledge.

Ghee and the Spine

The diya or the lamp in Indian philosophy signifies knowledge and the end of darkness that comes with fear. When the wick of this lamp is made from ghee, it stands upright through its burning time. The same thing happens to your spine – when you eat ghee, it stands upright. The fat is a terrific lubricant and gives the spine stability and strength. Now without a stable spine, think of what happens to the poor weight-bearing joints – hips, knees, ankles. And that's why not just pregnant women, even pehelwans across India consumed a lot of ghee (up to a litre a day). After all, pehelwani meant strength and without a strong spine there is no strength to show. Isn't that what you learn in your pilates class too? The importance of the core? Without a strong spine, you will always, always have a bulging tyre for a stomach. You want a flat stomach, you go *ghrutam pibet*.

The Ghee, Gut and Brain Connection

It's not just the lack of strength but also the lack of probiotic bacteria that's giving you that tyre which squeezes up from the top of your jeans. It also gives you unpredictable motions, sometimes mornings, sometimes evenings, sometimes nothing, sometimes running, sometimes constipated. Especially if you are a resident of Mumbai, Delhi, Bengaluru or Chennai and take morning flights to other metros. Then you pucca suffer, if not because of your stomach then because of the passenger next to you who couldn't go to the loo because of the stress of the morning flight.

Sorry guys, if I am not being sarcastic, I have to be gross. And while I am at it, let me tell you that the biggest problem of fad diets is not that they don't work but that they ruin the diversity and strength of your gut bacteria. I have been privy to too many burps and farts of absolutely stunning women who could have seen exactly how beautiful they look if only they had not opted for crash dieting, exotic health spas or procedures under the knife in their efforts to get pretty. That's because there is such a thing as 'gut bacteria and the brain axis', and when the strength and diversity of the good bacteria is diminishing so does the brain's ability to function optimally or be reasonable.

People who are always on some diet or the other have gut bacteria that resemble long-stay hospital patients and then every sensory organ starts functioning at below optimum including your brain. *Wajan kam nahi hota* but listening, sight, smell, skin, health *sab kam ho jata hai*. What a poor deal we cut ourselves for weight loss. All the while not even knowing that ghee, the way it is made at home, is not just good for maintaining the diversity and strength of the gut bacteria and spine but also makes for a potent fat-loss aid. The SCFA in ghee is now recognized as a 'pre-biotic', something which creates an environment conducive for the gut-friendly bacteria to prosper. That's also what makes it a great anti-allergen.

Fat-burning Coffee

A recent fad is to add a big blob of fat to your coffee so that your fat-burning picks up. Comes from the same funda that addition of essential fats will reduce the glycemic index. By the way, even the butter chai and arak (fermented barley spirit) of Spiti and Ladakhi societies are served with ghee. Easier assimilation and steady release of blood sugar.

Fact vs Fiction

Fiction	Fact
Ghee is fattening	Ghee by nature is lipolytic – it breaks down fat. And this is due to its unique SCFA structure.
Ghee is a saturated fat	It's a saturated fat, yes, but a unique one. It not just burns preferentially as fuel inside your body but actually helps mobilize fats from stubborn fat areas. Not like the unhealthy fats you find in your biscuits, cakes, pizza, etc.

Fiction	Fact
Ghee will increase cholesterol	Ghee reduces cholesterol by increasing the contribution of lipids to metabolism. The liver produces excess cholesterol under stress. Ghee helps you de-stress, sleep better and wake up fresher.
Ghee is harmful for the heart	Rich in antioxidants, conjugated linoleic acid (CLA) and fat-soluble vitamins like A, E, D, ghee has just what you need for a healthy heart.
Fine, ghee is good, but must not eat it too much	Traditionally, we add ghee to each meal. The quantity at which the taste of food is best is the right quantity. Only your tongue and stomach can tell you that, for example preparations like puran-poli need more than dal–chawal. 3–5 tsp a day is a good start.

Stepwise Instructions for Making Ghee

(As told by my mother and documented by my sister)

White butter

1. Skim the cream (malai) from the top of the milk daily. Store this in a ceramic or stainless steel vessel in the freezer. Do this every day for

a few days till the vessel is almost full. Keep this vessel full of cream in a cool, dry place till it thaws and reaches room temperature.

2. The next step is to warm the cream slightly so that the temperature is optimum to add dahi (culture). The trick is to warm the cream but not heat it. You can just leave the cream vessel on a hot tava after you are done with making rotis.

3. Add a good quantity of dahi to the cream and stir it sufficiently so that the dahi is mixed well.

4. Leave it in a cool, dry corner of the kitchen to set overnight or for a few hours (depending on the weather, this time may vary). Allow the cream to set like dahi.

5. Transfer this cream dahi to a bigger vessel, add some water and churn it with an old-fashioned wooden churner (ravi). The to-and-fro motion of the churner at a low speed is considered ideal for the churning process. It retains the moisture and the low temperature doesn't break the fragile fatty acid bonds. Do not use a mixer.

6. Separate the butter from the buttermilk. Wash this butter a few times under running water. You now have white butter which is good for consumption by itself or as a raw material for making ghee. The buttermilk can be used to make kadhi or can be consumed as is.

Ghee

1. Take a thick-bottomed copper kadai. Heat on full flame for 5–10 minutes till the butter melts and then on a low flame till the melted butter starts looking clear and there is a deposit of the ghee residue at the bottom of the kadai.

2. To check when the ghee is done is tricky and needs an expert eye. One way of checking this is to add 3–4 drops of water when the ghee is boiling. If it sizzles and splutters, it means the ghee is done.

3. Switch off the heat and allow the ghee to cool. It is necessary to do this to check if the ghee has been cooked perfectly.

4. The perfect ghee when cooled is whitish yellow

in colour and granular in texture (danedar).
If it's waxy, it means it's undercooked, and if
it's brown and granular, it's overcooked. If the
ghee is undercooked, you can boil it once again
and cook it further.

5. Pass the ghee through a sieve and store in a
closed container (not plastic).

Note

1. To get 1 kg of ghee it takes roughly 28 litres
of milk. It is the most distilled form of dairy
fat and contains nutrients of the richest grade.
And because of this it is safe for people who
are otherwise lactose intolerant.

2. Get desi cow milk to get all the benefits of
ghee. If not a desi cow, the next best option is
desi buffalo. Can't make ghee from tetra pack
or low-fat milk. Support goshalas by buying
their milk or ghee. They work not just in
cow protection but also promote sustainable
farming methods.

3. Indians abroad can:
   - buy organic milk from free grazing cows (or raw milk if available)
   - make it from white unsalted organic butter
   - or buy from goshalas or yoga stores

How to Have Ghee

The versatility of ghee is nothing short of miraculous.

1. Have a headache or sinus? Apply ghee on top of your head, massage it with a flat hand and watch the congestion disappear.

2. Have trouble sleeping or you snore or are depressed? Take a drop of ghee on your little finger and massage the insides of your nostrils.

3. Nightmares, bloated or plain sleepless – massage ghee on the soles of your feet till your palm feels warm and you'll sleep like a baby.

4. Eating something heavy? Puran-poli, biryani, dal baati? Load it up with ghee and see how it enhances taste, prevents overeating and leaves you feeling not just light but fulfilled.

5. Have heart health issues but feel like a bhajjiya, poori, vada? Fikar not. Deep-fry in homemade

ghee. With its high smoke point, it is the most potent antioxidant on earth. The main problem with deep-frying is polymerization or breakage of carbon bonds within the fatty acid chain. No such risk with ghee.

6. Skin breakouts with or before every period – eat ghee at least three times a day and feel glorious not just in your skin but even with the way the stomach feels, flat.

7. Struggling with weak joints or feet swelling post every flight? It's ghee again, either on roti or rice or simply by itself to keep the joints in good health.

8. Wanna kiss but the mouth stinks? Start and end your day by applying ghee to your teeth and gums and kiss your bleeding gums bye-bye.

9. Sneeze, burp or wake up farting every morning or simply too drunk from last night or jet lagged and have a meeting to attend – 1 tsp ghee with a pinch of kalanamak, drink it up with warm water and you will feel fresh like sunshine.

10. Wanna remember all the goodness of ghee but tend to forget and fall for the next fad? Eat ghee again. According to Ayurveda, it nourishes the tissues of the brain. Has a fatty acid composition that crosses the blood–brain barrier and ensures that you forget only what is not worth remembering. And that, ladies and gentlemen, is step one to happiness.

2

Kokum
The Natural Antacid

'Ahhh!' screamed my client's six-year-old in joy, tears streaming down her eyes. She had just tasted a ripe kokum for the first time in her life and was crying in response to its tangy, zesty taste. Kokum just knocks you out. It's rare for the palate to taste a flavour quite like it. Like the fragrance of the rose, it must be experienced as words cannot describe it. I thought I will save it for the end but will just say it, I use kokum to train the palate of the kids I work with and over a period of time they become naturally averse to chocolates and colas. Works well for all parties involved.

The kokum fruit (*Garcinia indica*) is blood-red in colour. It looks really beautiful and that's why the tree is used for ornamental purposes. To make it sound exotic, we could call it the forgotten fruit of the coast, but truth be told it still has a small local market and an emerging global market. It finds mention in the Vedas, *Arthashastra* and *Charaka Samhita* for both its good looks and its therapeutic properties. But sadly it is now in the list of NUS – Neglected and Underutilized Species – of the United Nations Food and Agriculture Organization (UNFAO). This recognition is almost an entry point for indigenous food to enter the European Union as a novel food. That's food which the Europeans have not been exposed to before 1997 but has evidence of being safe, beneficial in fact, for human consumption.

Our blood naturally maintains a pH of 7.4 which is slightly alkaline. However, our sedentary (more like lazy) lifestyle has made us prone to not just diabesity but also to acidity. It won't be an exaggeration to say that most urban folk have acidity, headaches and poor sleep for at least two days if not four days a week. We then tend to take a whole load of antacids, laxatives and even antibiotics to deal with the problems. All this abuse washes away our microbiome, the diverse societies of bacteria that live in our gut and promote our well-being. The 100 trillion bacteria that live in our gut can weigh up to a kilo or a little more. And these, as science is now discovering, are playing a huge role in the diseases of the rich, and I am not only talking of diabetes or heart disease but of the vitamin B12 and vitamin D deficiency that we all seem to be living with.

The thing with the microbiome ecosystem is that each of us has a unique one. It changes according to region, climate, genes and even diet. For example, vegetarians have an ecosystem that is different from that of the meat eaters, Asians have a gut microbiome which is far more equipped to break down lactose from milk than Caucasians' and rural and urban populations have clearly different strains of bacteria too. Our changing lifestyles also compromise the naturally rich, diverse gut ecosystem. Eating out every week, late lunches and onslaught of coffee during meetings ruin not just our health but also the health of these symbiotic partners. When our bacterial ecosystem is compromised, our ability to pick up or assimilate nutrients from food is compromised too. Almost everyone who has low B12 or D levels has enough food on the plate but is handicapped by impaired absorption of nutrients, a function of acid-base balance in the body. A weakened biosystem also disturbs the pH or creates acidity in the body.

Acidity and Vitamin D

If you have had too many antacids, or proton inhibitors as they are called, your ability to pick up not just vitamin B12 but vitamin D and even minerals like calcium and magnesium is seriously reduced. Almost everyone with acidity will complain of teeth or bone trouble, and one of the reasons is impaired calcium absorption. You will suffer from acidity, headaches or flatulence and even your sleep will go for a toss due to

---

impaired vitamin D absorption. In fact, you can think of vitamin D as a hormone, one that your skin produces on sun exposure, with the help of gut-friendly bacteria. Vitamin D plays a crucial role in sleep, ensuring that you hit the restorative sleep stage and that all your recovery hormones are able to carry out their repair and maintenance work. There is emerging evidence in medicine to suggest that vitamin D pathways may be linked to gut homeostasis, or maintenance of the ecosystem. And vitamin D levels affect the signalling between microbes and their host, we humans.

The Miracle in Kokum

Kokum is perhaps more necessary today than ever. It has been celebrated for its ability to keep acidity at bay, thus ensuring that you maintain not just a good acid-base balance but with it a harmonious ecosystem for microbiota. And microbes reside not just in our gut but in every orifice of the body. From the ears to the anus, from the vagina to the nostrils, every single opening will have its share of friendly bacteria. They cause no harm, help in every way, feed off you and in return protect you, the classical symbiotic relationship we read about in our biology textbooks.

Little wonder then that kokum is used as a healing herb for ulcers, ear infection, common cold and even UTI (urinary tract infection). Traditionally, it's grandma's go-to herb to cure acidity, bloating and flatulence. It's something that you would reach out for in the kitchen when you have overeaten or underslept or are just plain under the weather.

Kokum was known to smoothen digestion and therefore it has been used in every possible way in Indian kitchens – from flavouring agent to pickle to sherbet. Better digestion essentially means better assimilation of nutrients and effective elimination of toxins, thus maintaining both the pH and the diversity of the microbiome ecosystem. This ensures better breakdown of nutrients in food, be it vitamin B12 or the elusive vitamin D. While vitamin B12 plays a role in the absorption of iron and production of red blood cells, it also keeps the homocysteine levels in check. High homocysteine levels are linked to low fertility and high blood pressure levels. It could be precisely for these reasons that Ayurveda celebrates kokum for its ability to regulate menses and to protect the heart, *ek teer se do nishaane*.

Vitamin D on the other hand is integral to sleep quality, the functioning of the thyroid and parathyroid glands and even in the absorption and assimilation of calcium, making kokum a traditional medicine even for rheumatism. One that works at reducing inflammation in the joints and even helps strengthen the bone mineral density – one stone, two birds.

And There's Much More

Garcinol, the most active ingredient in kokum, is an anti-bacterial, anti-viral and antioxidant agent. It's for this reason that kokum is considered a functional food, that is, food (not pill or capsule) which besides having nutrients also possesses health benefits and disease prevention properties. The ORAC value – oxygen radical absorption capacity, a measure of the antioxidant score of any food – of kokum is very high. No wonder it is now used in a whole range of cosmetic applications from lotions for cracked heels to lipsticks. Multiple studies have shown that garcinol from kokum suppresses carcinogenesis (growth of cancer) by inhibiting the enzymes that promote the growth of cancerous cells. Garcinol's role in cellular apoptosis (cellular death) and its effect on cancer could even provide an alternative therapy for cancer.

It could well be for this reason that this magical red fruit is often called amrut (life enhancer) kokum in the land of its birth.

Hydroxyl citric acid (HCA) is a characteristic ingredient of kokum which is a well-known weight-loss aid. One that regulates appetite and optimizes fat-burning, and occupies an unchallenged position in every fat-burning pill out there. If you ever wanted *Garcinia cambogia* for its weight-loss effects, well, look no further than our own kokum for it is this same HCA that you find in kokum. Besides weight loss, HCA is also used to reduce cholesterol and anxiety, all three important for the typical urban lifestyle.

Kokum also has extremely high levels of **bio-flavonoids**, making it extremely useful as an anti-tumour agent, even better than curcumin or haldi.

How Kokum Is Used

The kokum fruit, also known as amsul, is used as a flavouring agent in dals and sabzis, to add just the right tanginess to the preparation. It has a very specific job in the preparation of sabzis like bhindi, which is to ensure that it doesn't get too sticky or tough to digest. While cooking suran, arbi and other tubers, it serves to inhibit the itch or irritation that these veggies can cause to the throat. In Assam it is used to make tangy fish curry called tenga.

You can also eat it raw like you eat kaccha aam, with some salt and masala. Crazy, zesty taste which also prevents cavities. Functional but fun.

Mixed with coconut milk, it is the key ingredient for the famed sol kadhi of the Western Ghats. So beautifully complex and integrated in flavours – it's the stuff that inspires Michelin star chefs.

Kokum agal or kokum water If you stylishly garnish water with lime, orange rind or pudina, know that kokum is the trendstarter. Called agal, this water is used to prevent dehydration, acidity or simply as a pick-me-up drink.

Kokum sherbet My absolute favourite. Mixed with sugar, spices, rock salt, this concentrate, popularly called amrut kokum, could just be the sweetest thing to drink your way to weight loss. With a fan base that ranges from Alia Bhatt to Anupam Kher, it's a drink that keeps small women cooperatives in business, makes stylishly cool shots and leaves you feeling truly light.

Kokum butter It nurtures and regenerates skin cells and therefore finds its way into cosmetics from foot creams to high-end hair conditioners. Farm festivals that promote local foods and food products often sell raw kokum butter in the form of small blocks and you can use it for many home beauty applications. Rubbing the soles of your feet with kokum butter just before going to bed will provide restful sleep to the most stressed-out mind.

3

Banana
The Recharger

Fruits are amazing, but if there is a first among equals, it's the banana. Among Maharashtrians, we have a tradition called oti bharna, a ritual where a woman is gifted some rice, coconut and fruits. At one time these gifts were all you needed for a full life – you sat with the pallu of your sari spread out on your lap and the elder women of the family or neighbourhood showered you with goodies. There are many occasions where one's oti gets bharaoed but the most popular one is during the seventh month of pregnancy or baby shower.

So, as the woman gets full-blown pregnant and enters the last trimester, she receives the customary rice, coconut, seasonal fruits and all the stuff she's craving for. There's one thing, however, that's not allowed and that is the banana. A banana plant can only give birth once, you see. The banana fruit receives everything from the tree and after that the plant doesn't reproduce any more. Very different from the mango or jamun tree, for example, where year after year they can blossom into new flowers that turn into fruits. The *one child* policy existed in nature even before China conceptualized it. Now in India we first ask girls when they will marry, after that we ask them when they will give good news, and while still pregnant with the good news, we want to know when the next one will arrive. So the banana is not gifted to tell the woman to have more than one child! Oh boy! Subtle and how?

It's interesting to see how things interplay when we are more connected to the earth, how subtle, manipulative and fun messages can be sent with just a fruit. But that apart, the banana is the super fruit, super for kids, super for athletes, and if you are a Karisma Kapoor fan or simply a fan of how fit she has looked through the years, her secret is simply the banana.

The banana was always regarded as special in our culture. No matter where you hail from, the pooja mandap will always be decorated with banana stumps and every sooji halwa or sheera that's offered as prasad will have a ripe banana mixed in it.

Then came the post-Second-World-War era and the meaning of everything from food to health changed. The banana is now a fattening fruit that must be avoided if you have diabesity (the twin burden of obesity and diabetes which is seen as the world's big disease) or simply any other hormonal disorder. It's like the rumour mills are churning overtime to malign the poor fruit. But is everything that is said about the banana really true? Must one really avoid it if one is trying to lose weight or regulate blood sugar or blood pressure? Well, all I can say is that there are lies and then there are lies. And everything that the weight-loss world has told you about the banana is untrue.

Have You Had a True Indian Banana?

Broadly, there are three types of bananas found in the region – the big green ones, the small yellow ones called the elaichi banana and the medium-size red ones. Unfortunately, the native green bananas have almost disappeared from our cities, replaced by the giant yellow ones that you get everywhere in the world. The small yellow ones still survive and the red ones – the red ones are the like the rare, precious pieces of art understood and appreciated by a really tiny following. Each one of the native species is beautiful but the one that really needs your support is the sukeli. Mostly produced by the East Indian community that is struggling not just to keep up its identity and language but also its food traditions. Sukeli is the sun-dried banana (looks like churros) with a peculiar sweetness that comes from being sun-dried in a basket that not just helps retain the moisture but also increases the shelf life of fruit. It is eaten both as a delicacy and as an immunity booster.

The Miracle of the Banana

The banana is packed with all the nutrients you need for a quick recharge. You have probably seen tennis players munch on the fruit in between sets, only to return with that ace serve and win the games. It could be the potassium, the vitamin B6 or its low to medium glycemic index or it could simply be the fact that all this goodness comes together to make the banana so special, almost as if nature packed and sealed all its performance-aiding nutrients in a tiny, tiny package. The potassium ensures that blood pressure doesn't rise and that your intra- and extracellular environment is equipped to quickly expel all the metabolic waste. The vitamin B6 is a metabolism enhancer and prevents brain fatigue from setting in. The fibre and the low glycemic index of the banana ensure that blood sugar rises in a slow, steady rate so there's no risk of a slump unlike a caffeine/nicotine energy fix. The banana is simply the best snack you can have for yourself any time of the day, the ultimate accessory in your handbag.

And that's not all. It also:

1. Is nature's own stomach-soother. From diarrhoea to constipation to IBS to everything in between, the fruit works at improving your gut health. The pre-biotic is at work here, yes, the one you will find in fancy bottles online, but nothing comes close to this natural beauty.

2. Strengthens bones. The minerals, the electrolytes and fibre help not just the bone mineral density but can positively reduce menstrual cramps too.

3. Beats the blues. Nursing a broken heart or been backstabbed by a colleague, chew on a banana. The vitamin B6 and the magnesium will help you find it in your heart to forgive them and move on.

Fact vs Fiction

Fiction	Fact
It is high on sugar	Nope. It's all natural sugar in the form of fructose and comes loaded with vitamin B. Always remember, the trick with sugar is to take it in naturally occurring forms
Avoid if you are diabetic	With a low to medium glycaemic index, the banana is not just safe but even recommended by the American Diabetic Association for its multiple health benefits
Avoid if you have blood pressure	Naturally high in electrolytes, it makes for a great mid-meal snack, especially when you feel that you are coming down with a throbbing headache.
Avoid if you want a flat stomach	Rich in fibre and pectin, it allows for a good build-up of healthy bacteria which in turn reduces your chances of looking or feeling bloated
It's fattening	Give me a break. Real low on fat but magically carries some plant sterol that not just helps fat-burning but even prevents plaquing of arteries and reduces cholesterol. Go to hell, yucky oats.

Fiction	Fact
Okay but I am trying to lose weight	Then nothing better than this God's own fruit. High in vitamin B6, minerals and fibre, this is one fruit that will pull you out of this frustration of losing weight and fill you with enthusiasm for workouts and it won't let you go mad for a pastry or chocolate.

How to Eat It

One of the things that define superfoods is the many ways in which we can eat them and the various ways they aid us. The banana is especially versatile:

Banana stem Makes for a great sabzi, especially when mixed with some lentils. If we could, we should send it as India's official entry to win the award for the most creative use of pulses to celebrate the UNFAO's Year of Pulses 2016. A delicacy both in the South and in the East, the stem is truly special and medicinal. Traditionally, papads were made by mixing the atta only with water that had been passed through the banana stem so that a good balance of electrolytes was maintained. Little wonder then that Ayurveda recognizes the stem for its ability to heal the kidneys. So how does this sound to you: if you continued eating traditionally, you could have the papad and keep the kidneys (and the heart, blood pressure, etc.) happy too.

Banana leaf To start with, you could simply eat on a banana leaf. In fact, every time you serve food on a banana leaf, the food gets its own distinct flavour. This comes from the polyphenols on the banana leaf – they not just up the antioxidant value of the meal but also ensure that blood sugars climb in a slow, steady rate. It may seem unreal but if you routinely feel dead tired after lunch or are struggling to go off the ciggy post lunch, just switch to eating on a banana leaf. It's eco-friendly too.

Raw bananas From chips to bhaaji to flour, the raw banana will lend itself to every mood you are in. The chips are a great snack, the bhaaji is yummy and the flour will make you feel very virtuous as it is gluten-free. A part of every Indian's diet in one way or the other, the dry banana is also a source of the amino acid tryptophan. Tryptophan is linked with multiple positives, from reducing mood swings to giving you good sleep. And I say, girl, this is just what you need when you get all worked up over PMS or when you want to heal a heartbreak. Now you know why you reach out instinctively for kela chips when you are pissed.

The ripe banana zaroor khana. The first fruit that your tongue tasted, your stomach digested and your colon excreted will work for you till the very end. And while at it, it will ease your nerves with vitamin B6, strengthen your capillaries and bones with minerals and your gut with its pectin and soluble fibre. Never before in the history of mankind has come a fruit so popular, cutting across classes, masses, continents. I have always felt that if only five-star hotels in India provided the local banana instead of the California apple in the room, the hotel guests would not just be a happier but even a thinner lot. But then who wants to give and, more important, take fukat advice. You can eat the banana first thing in the morning, after exercise, in between studies, flights and even fights.

It's one of the only three fruits that's an exception to the rule of 'don't eat fruits with your meals', the other two being jackfruit and mango. Banana, ghee, sugar with milk and chapatti is a popular Maharashtrian lunch item for school kids called shikran. Your South Indian mami with mogra in her hair will love her banana post-lunch as much as she loves her degree kapi in the morning. Versatile, remember, eat it in your style, the banana is all yours.

Banana flower Swear, it's a real thing. So local and so so exotic that it doesn't even have a global name. It's typically turned into a sabzi and is popular from the north-east to the south of India and everywhere in between. Like the mother it is known by different names in different regions but is usually mixed with seeds rich in essential fats and protein, like peanuts, kaju, til, etc., to produce a delicious sabzi. In Bengali cuisine, the mochar (Bengali for the banana flower) ghanto, a dry preparation with potatoes and coconut, is a lunch delicacy. If you are struggling with low haemoglobin levels, break-outs and acne or simply are hitting menopause, this is the vegetable you want.

The flower takes a long time to peel and is a work of not just patience but skill, but it will wash away every hormonal sin out there.

So remember, dar ke aage banana hai, and banana zaroor khana hai.

4

Kaju
The Antidepressant

'We associate health with food, instead of agriculture, that's why we get it wrong,' said Anna Lartey, director of the UNFAO. If there's a single sentence that sums up the ideas in this book, it's this. Agriculture is about growing what is suitable for the region and then eating it in the right season. It also means that there are versatile and varied ways to consume that food, not just by humans but by other living beings in that region, which results in less waste and makes it more sustainable. Because such food is local, it's more traditional and traditional, means that it will have varied therapeutic applications.

Among the nuts, the humble kaju has always had a bad rep. Almonds and walnuts are great for the heart; however, the kaju apparently causes cholesterol and is fattening. The kaju, though, is not really the type of fruit to get worked up over small misunderstandings. Rich in vitamin B6 and folate, this nut is forgiving and simply wants to inform you that, since you have a liver, you are the one producing the cholesterol. After all, it is only a plant, not some animal or dreadful human that it can produce cholesterol. But it does have a beautiful profile of fatty acids and phytosterols that have a wide range of biological activity in the human body ranging from anti-inflammatory to antibacterial, antioxidative to anti-cancerous.

You are avoiding it because the fashion magazine food writer is making the same mistake that your dietician is making, who is making the same mistake that your doctor is making, by not putting agriculture in the same bracket as health, as Anna Lartey pointed out.

And if you did put the two in the same bracket, you would realize that it's not about eating the Mediterranean diet, it's about eating your traditional diet. Because if you are a numbers-driven person, the number of obese in the Mediterranean would boggle you. Then you would stumble upon the next big thing called the Nordic diet, only to realize that the government and the stakeholders in that region are promoting the local food and eating habits because they have realized that it's not about being on the Med diet but about creating food systems that deliver good nutrition to the present and future generations in a sustainable manner. Because local is traditional and traditional is sustainable (local plants and crops are climate-change-resilient). And sustainability matters because the way we are going, climate change is going to kill us before heart attack does.

We are, however, a country where kaju is local but it is oats from some packet (again, consider your carbon footprint) that is recognized as good for cholesterol. It is at least three times richer in iron than spinach but it doesn't find a mention in our school textbooks. Cashew fruit or apple as it is called has at least five times more vitamin C than orange but you won't learn that in school and the government doesn't give a damn if some orange juice brands itself as vitamin C rich while the poor cashew farmer doesn't know how to make cash from his crop. Then a global cola giant walks in and says, hey! we will buy that cashew apple and make it into a juice. We will package it, rebrand it, the farmer still won't make money, the consumer will still stay fat from eating industrialized food and we will still earn huge profits. And all is well with the world.

Olives and Avocados

Take the case of the olive: we eat olives or use olive oil for heart health but what about kaju? You will find more people eating avocado salad in Mumbai than the number of people who have even heard of, forget eaten, cashew sprouts. Now avocado, like olives, is not local. So anywhere in India, especially in Mumbai, a kaju would travel a smaller distance to land on your plate than would olives or avocado. Fewer food miles mean smaller agricultural footprint – that would mean you are one of those really, really smart global citizens who take pride in local food. So all in all, it's not about the olive or the avocado (by the way, in the 1960s they were trying to tell Greece to get off the olive and have vegetable oils) but about figuring out that local food has value and is richer in micronutrients even if schools don't teach it, health professionals are unaware of it and governments don't have policies for it.

So why the big bhashan? Because I am eating kaju and feeling generous and you should know the facts, man. You can't be sitting at your doctor's table with a cholesterol report in your hand, listening to how you can eat walnuts and almonds, but cannot touch kaju. So here's the lowdown on this super-nut.

Basically, if you are losing sleep at night and

spend the day feeling anxious and dead tired, this is the nut that you need to crack. Its amino acid profile, minerals and vitamins could well be the inspiration behind the 'stay calm and get on' line of posters. The amino acids help, among other things, in the production of serotonin, the natural sleeping pill whose only side effect is a stable, happy mood the next day.

Rujuta's Cashew Milk

Soak 4–5 cashews in a bit of milk for 4–5 hours. Then pour the milk and cashew in a pestle and pound it. Top this nutty milk mixture with more milk. Add sugar to taste and some saffron if you want. Drink cold or hot just before going to bed. You will never have more fun sleeping alone.

Magnesium is essential for nerves to relax. The next time you are PMSing and want to kill someone or just die crying, just chill and chew some cashew or if your husband is officially middle-aged and wakes up in the middle of the night with a cramping calf, let him munch on cashew too. Its tryptophan (an amino acid) and vitamin B combination is leading to an ever-increasing interest in using kaju as a natural antidepressant. Watch this space.

Fact vs Fiction

Like all superfoods, cashew of course works double time and has a whole lot of other uses. It is rich in copper, iron, vitamin E. More on this below:

Fiction	Fact
Avoid if you have cholesterol	Its phytosterols and stanols will not just reduce the LDL and help improve HDL but also reduce absorption of cholesterol from the small intestine. Overall bad news for pharma companies selling statins, if you start eating cashews.

Fiction	Fact
Avoid if you have a heart condition	Mineral- and vitamin-rich, especially vitamin E, cashew works as an anti-ageing agent and is particularly good for heart conditions. Prevents plaque build-up and lowers blood pressure, two big precursors of heart disease. Cashew also has copper, which is vital to keep your blood vessels in working order.
Avoid if you are losing weight	Never has there been a bigger lie than this. Rich in vitamin B, critical for carbohydrate metabolism and for ensuring that you never reach that dreaded weight-loss plateau.
Avoid if you are diabetic	Low glycaemic index, rich in essential fatty acids, rich in fibre, if cashews are not anti-diabetic then nothing is.
Avoid if have PCOD or hypothyroidism	Great source of iron, prevents adult acne, a sign of hormonal imbalance, improves fertility and works like a diuretic. Need I say more?

How to Eat Cashews

Leaves Chew on them, or boil them in water and gargle with it. Great for oral health.

Fruit Ranging from yellow to fleshy pink to bright orange, thanks to its anthocyanins and carotenes, a class of antioxidants, the fruit is a great source of vitamin C and an excellent immunity booster. It works like magic in getting rid of oral ulcers and cavities and is especially good for chronic ulcerative colitis or to ease a bloated stomach.

Tender cashews Now you got to be a real Konkan person like me to even know that there is such a thing. Passed on like a secret potion from grandfathers to their granddaughters, this is one delicacy valued higher than gold. From the flawless skins that signify high fertility levels to the gut microbiota diversity that it builds, you can blame the classic Konkani heart of gold that goes with a caustic tongue on this one. Come on, indulge me, it costs you nothing. Eaten like an usal or sondal or the way you would make rajma, this is had with rice. This is easily the best tasting complete plant protein on earth, and for those who like it all free, its gluten-free, lactose free and vegan too.

Cashews The most versatile of the lot. Have it like

a morning meal, crush it and add to your halwas and laddoos, chew on it when you are in meetings that are unnerving or on long flights that make you dull and bloated. Especially important when one is going through a hormonal transition like hitting puberty or menopause, or simply going through teenage or a rough break-up, the cashew really just helps you keep it together. It draws on this property from the tree which is planted on the coast to prevent soil erosion during floods and to keep the water table stable during droughts.

Neero The virgin juice of cashews which goes through an exotic process of being crushed under human feet, passing through a basin that is tied by a rope and collected under the tree in an earthen pot that is later buried in sand. Neero that's allowed to ferment just right and distilled turns to the beautiful, intoxicating and aromatic feni. Now someone needs to come up with a *Sideways* kind of movie so that we may fall in love with the process all over again and realize that our wine is actually our feni. Neero is just juice and you can have it, as a nice non-alcoholic drink or as an immunity enhancer. The feni you should get introduced to by a local aunty who will sit with you on the low bench outside her house, watching the world go by while telling you that the drink is given to children (tiny amounts of course: strong alcohol content) to accelerate recovery from illness. As for you and the aunty, middle age is a kind of illness too, one that can accelerate ageing if you don't hit the brakes on time. Feni is that brake, from improving gut microbiota diversity to the *halka halka suroor*, it will teach you that happiness lies in the middle and not in the extreme. Drink up.

5

Ambadi
The Stomach-Soother

If you have lived in India or have Indian roots you may have heard your grandma caution against eating green leafy vegetables during the monsoon. If you went to a school like the one I went to, you would probably dismiss this as superstition or some silly native practice. Modern education has it that green leafy veggies, especially spinach, are rich in iron and that meals should be colourful.

Ayurveda, on the other hand, teaches us that eating should be tweaked according to the season. And that one should not eat what will disturb one's personal constitution or even the universe at large. It is based on the belief that what is harmful to the pinda (person) also harms the brahmanda (the entire creation).

The monsoon period is called Chaturmasa or the four months when the lord of creation, Bramha, goes into overdrive. Vishnu, the preserver, on the other hand, sleeps.

Along with green leafy vegetables, meat eating, more specifically fish eating, is given up during this time too. This is based on the principles of sustainability. Fish breed during the monsoon, and if you wish to eat enough fish in this lifetime and leave behind enough for your grandchildren, you give up eating fish during this period. Not such a bad idea then, don't you agree?

It's the same for green leafy veggies as they are a breeding ground for microorganisms which are also under the sway of Lord Brahma's creative overdrive, making not just them but even the meat of the livestock that feeds on them unsafe for human consumption. The exception to this rule are a few local greens the queen of which is ambadi.

Ancient Is the New Modern

Where do you get your iron and protein from if green veggies and meat are not allowed during these four months? Fikar not, for you can always fall back on the grains. This is when some really interesting meals are traditionally eaten to get a good profile of essential fatty acids, amino acids, fibre and phytonutrients.

It's the time to prepare khichdis and kheers from bajra and jowar, basically local millet. And to consume them along with some papads that you made in summer. And if only we followed this ritual, our NRI cousin wouldn't be the one to introduce us to the ancient grain pops while shopping in a US mall.

But as I've said too often in this book, the poor man's food (always a representation of native eating habits) from one continent becomes the rich man's weight-loss aid in another continent.

Till the advent of kale, this was pretty much one-way traffic. For the first time, a poor European farmer's winter food went to the rest of the world. It is now indiscriminately juiced, sliced, diced and eaten in all seasons from Bengaluru to Bangkok to Boston as healthy, detox, weight loss, whatever. There's even a sequence in *Modern Family* where Mitch fills in Cam on the latest gossip and announces that kale is the new spinach. PS: Please watch *Modern Family* if you haven't.

The Miracle in Ambadi

The green-leaved, red-stemmed ambadi belongs to the hibiscus family of plants, taller than the other greens and more acidic (which is why it is not affected by the microorganisms during monsoons). It's eaten all over the country and known by many different names. Ambadi is its Marathi name; in Telugu it is called gongura and famously turned into a delicious pickle; in English it is known as the roselle plant. Whatever its name, it is one of our most extraordinary plants.

India is a gene-rich country: our agricultural research scientists have recorded at least 1532 edible plants. Tribals are a repository of this plant knowledge, and they use these plants as food, medicine and sources of income. Ambadi is the tribal woman's source of folic acid and iron. Easy to digest and cook, it is also without the side effects of constipation that come with an iron pill. Most important, it is high in slowly digestible starch, making it an excellent vegetable to sustain and nurture the gut ecosystem. The rains come with their share of stomach infections and this invariably leads to loss of good bacteria from the system. Now, how wonderful is the traditional food system which encourages diversity even in the greens you eat?

Just 1 per cent of 1532 edible plants would mean 15, so my question to you is how many native plants do you eat? We keep eating the same baingan, gobi, aloo, bhindi. And if we eat out we go for broccoli, mushroom, rucola and the likes. Our apathy towards our local greens has earned them the tag of **orphan crops**: the ones that no one wants to eat and therefore no one wants to grow. And this is sad because local greens, like ambadi, are climate-resilient, grow in every condition, need no labour and can bring relatively easy income for our farmers.

So my free advice to you is that you should be eating at least 0.5 per cent of these indigenous plants. That's because a diet rich in diverse vegetarian sources of foods is low on TMAO, a type of bacterial metabolite that's found in our body and is linked to atherosclerosis (plaquing of arteries, bad news for the heart). Low diversity in vegetarian sources leads to poor diversity in the microbiome ecosystem in the gut. As food science now knows, this can accelerate ageing, lead to depression and has a high pro-inflammatory potential – so overall bad news for health and weight loss.

Tribals use ambadi to build more strength in the stomach, improve immunity and prevent diarrhoea. It's time we re-adopt this vegetable in our lives – it will keep adults in urban societies free from irritable bowel syndrome (IBS) and depression, and help our kids fight frequent illness and allergies.

Another notable factor here is that the ambadi bhaji or sabzi is always eaten with fibrous bhakris made of makai, jowar, bajra or ragi and these traditional food combos make for low glycemic index meals. Essentially this means lesser risk of non-communicable diseases like diabetes, obesity, cancer, etc. Patronizing local food systems allows for sustainability not just of our ecology but also or our blood sugar regulatory mechanism.

Cuba is one of the few countries trying to do its bit to spread awareness of the benefits of eating more diverse vegetables. Their municipalities have to compulsorily have urban and peri-urban agriculture and their media, both TV and radio, have to participate in their public policies. Which means that there can be no advertisements of unhealthy food. Now imagine Indian TV with no ads of instant noodles, chocolates, colas, etc. And municipalities that make it compulsory for builders to mark farm plots per flat versus parking lot per flat. Oh boy, I am just loving it! ;)

There are ambadi and ambadi-like 'spinaches' in every part of India, devoured by the elders, shunned by the young. The time for them to return is now. Kale is nothing but someone else's ambadi, someone who lives 5000 miles away from you. And the thing with food is that the more it travels, the more it loses its nutrients. There's a catchy term for it – food miles. And the longer the food travels to land in your plate, the longer your navel travels away from your spine. Hello paunch, bye-bye washboard abs. Don't like the name ambadi? Call it roselle, okay?

How to Eat Ambadi

Flowers Ambadi has these beautiful red flowers and a bhagat (a doctor in tribal communities) will boil them in water and give it to people fighting stomach ailments. The West uses roselle tea as a hangover remedy or simply as a detox drink and an alternative to caffeine drinks. Europe is a big consumer of this drink and it is part of many herbal and yoga teas.

Leaves Eaten as a delicacy from Meghalaya to Tamil Nadu, it's among the only green leafy vegetables eaten in the monsoon and all the way up to the winter when more greens like palak and sarson become available. It turns into delicious sabzis that are eaten with fibre-rich millets, to curries that are offered to Mahalakshmi, the goddess of wealth, and Andhra has a speciality dish where it is cooked with gosht. As a good source of minerals like iron, vitamin B and folic acid, there is now renewed interest in the leaf as an anti-carcinogen.

Stems Eaten and cooked along with the sabzi. Can also turn into ropes. Or you could use the fibre to make a mat, and if you are one of those sustainability or organic architects who trip on all things Pondicherry, you could even turn them into blocks and use them as sound-proofing material. Tribals will use this as a sieve, or make a jhadoo out of it and even fabric. But these are almost extinct arts now.

Seeds Crushed and turned into oil, extensively used for lighting lamps and can even be used for cooking. Currently being looked into as a biodiesel too.

Basically, ambadi has everything that makes it a cool food item. It is extremely versatile and all it needs is some IIT or IIM gang to come up with a start-up idea where local produce is patronized by celeb chefs and marketed as boutique or niche in high-end restaurants. And then the ambadi won't be so orphaned any more, small farmers will make money and start-ups will finally go beyond the low-cal health food delivery systems.

6

Rice
The Grain That Sustains

'You think he is not coming and eating because he's on a diet?' whispered my friend in my ear. Her friend's father-in-law had passed away and it was his tenth day. As per tradition, a mound of rice was being offered to the father-in-law. If the crow, in whose form the FIL was supposed to come, pecked at the rice, then it would mean that he had led a fulfilling life and would continue his journey towards mukti. If not, as in this case, it meant that he would be reborn to fulfil unfulfilled wishes. 'Shit! Uncleji is coming back to lose those last five kilos,' my friend concluded. The level of jokes is falling everywhere, not just on prime time comedy shows. And losing weight is a burden you carry even after you die.

As I walked back home, I thought of the now dead father-in-law. When he was born, his parents must have written his name on rice at his naming ceremony. During Bhai Dooj, his sisters must have put a tikka on his forehead with some water so that the grains of rice would stick. When he got married, every guest must have showered the couple with rice. When he entered his new home, his wife must have kicked a pot of rice as a gesture of homecoming and to ward off the evil eye. From birth to death, rice shadows you in every big and small moment and then post-fifty, when you turn diabetic, it's taken off your plate, just like that.

Ayurveda celebrates rice as the symbol of health, wealth and fertility and that's why, from newborns to newly-weds to new acquisitions, everything gets showered with rice. Rice is the first grain that you get introduced to. You get off an exclusive breast milk diet and you get on to rice either in the form of pej or kanjee (rice soup) or really diluted rice itself. Of course it may have some ghee or salt and as you grow up to be eight or nine months there will even be some dal but the base is always rice. And there are many reasons for that, the most important being that it is suitable for people of all kinds of constitutions, doshas – vata, pitta and kapha. That's Sanskrit for non-allergen, gluten-free and high on the protein digestibility score. That's exactly why big or small, man or woman, happy or angry, constipated or running, rich or poor, rice is everybody's comfort food.

The Miracle in Rice: Lysine

Rice is almost the only grain to have high levels of an essential amino acid called lysine. All other grains and cereals are limited by this amino acid, which means lysine is either totally absent or is not present in adequate amounts in other grains. It's an essential amino acid, which means it cannot be produced by the body and has to be consumed through the food we eat. Now the big deal with lysine, or L-lysine as the body-building world calls it, is that it's a precursor to the human growth hormone (HGH).

HGH, secreted by the pituitary gland, peaks

at night and helps with the all-important repair and growth function of the body. By the time you are thirty, this goes into decline and is responsible for increase in adipose tissue, decrease in insulin sensitivity (hello diabesity), thinning of skin, loss of hair, etc. – in short, ageing.

When your stomach asks for rice at night, it's for the high levels of lysine and ease of digestibility. And feeding of essential amino acids at dinner allows the human growth hormone to peak optimally. So you wake up feeling lighter, take less time in the loo and actually even manage to get that workout done before office.

HGH is particularly important in the first eight years of your life when you reach a whole lot of growth milestones. So when dadi-nani say rice for your infant, they are saying more lysine, sweetie, fewer infections, better growth. Imagine a culture so rich that even without high-tech labs they knew that the infant needed something easy to digest, something to propel her growth, increase her height and improve her bone density.

Fact vs Fiction

Rice is a perfect example of the weight-loss industry (with the aid of 'research and marketing') brainwashing entire cultures into believing the food that they have always eaten is somehow harming them. Nutrition bodies, the world over, have recognized this phenomenon as 'nutrition transition', where ancient communities are becoming increasingly prone to diabetes, obesity, heart and other lifestyle diseases after switching from their local, seasonal foods to something exotic, non-native and mass produced.

Fiction	Fact
Rice has starch	Cooked rice has less than 10 per cent starch left Starch is a source of energy as it's converted to glucose in the body, so we need it
Rice has a high glycaemic index and is bad for diabetics	Rice is traditionally eaten with dal/sabzi/meat/dahi, etc., along with ghee, and this lowers the glycaemic index of meals and is therefore totally safe for diabetics. Bhutan is a predominantly

Fiction	Fact
	rice-eating country and has no problem of diabetes. So there is much more to diabetes than simply blaming it on rice.
Rice is carbs, so avoid, especially at night	No food is just carbs or proteins or fats Rice has crucial amino acids, vitamins and many phytonutrients along with carbs Carbs are essential for our body and have a calming effect; therefore, rice is great as a dinner option
Eat brown rice, not white	Traditionally, we have always eaten hand-pounded or single-polished rice which is white in colour, not brown This kind of rice contains just the optimum amount of fibre, not high, and lets the body assimilate all the nutrients from it, for example, vitamin B6 and zinc
Okay fine, rice is nice, but must not eat too much of it	Too much of hawa is also bad, so let go of your fear of rice, eat it and trust your tongue and stomach to guide you

How to Eat Rice

All traditional communities or cultures across the world eat the grain along with other food. This is a sensible, scientific method of eating rice – one that mixes rice with other legumes/pulses and fats like ghee so that the meal has a low GI and has the complete amino acid profile in a specific ratio. This is what the UNFAO calls future food – plant protein – a non-meat source that provides a complete amino acid profile and is easy to digest. Khichdi, for example – so simple and unassuming that it's easy to miss the science behind it.

Things We Don't Know about Rice

Rice:
- Promotes growth of probiotic bacteria, eases bowel movement and rids you of bloating
- Prevents premature wrinkling
- Supports good hair growth
- Has inositol, which has fat-burning, anti-anxiety and irritability-reducing properties

- Allows for better assimilation of vitamin D and calcium
- Is a good source of methionine, an amino acid required to break down fat in your liver

FAQs on Rice

Brown or white?

I come from a rice-farming family and know for a fact that growing rice is among the most extensive and magical processes. The brown rice that I referred to in my first book is the hand-pounded or single-polished rice that we made on our farms. It isn't like the brown rice in the market; in fact, it is much closer to white rice. Eating more than the required amount of fibre comes in the way of mineral absorption. That's exactly why women spend days together pounding the rice – to optimize the fibre by removing the excess (which gets fed to cattle – sustainability anyone?) and allows for better absorption of minerals from the meals you eat.

If you don't find hand-pounded or single-polished rice, you can eat white rice.

How to cook rice?

The best rice is the one that grows closest to where you reside, ideally from a small farm. So pick single-origin rice; packet rice can never give you the guarantee that it's from one farm, that all the grains matured together, etc. Cook your rice the way your grandma taught you to. There is no such thing as 'removing starch' from rice, that's an essential nutrient, along the molecules of which many nutrients reside. The method of 'removing water' from rice removes these anti-ageing nutrients. Traditionally 'removed water' would be cooked along with some grains and offered as kanji or pej to the oldest and the youngest members of the family as its easy on the gastrointestinal tract, is liquid so no need to chew much (you may either have not grown your teeth or lost your teeth) and the vitamin B helped in metabolic processes. So the removal of water came out of more intelligent use of resources and not from fear of getting fat. Eating rice at night is a brilliant strategy for those who plan to but don't work out in the morning, as it can really help with restorative sleep.

Which rice to eat?

There are more than a thousand varieties of rice in India, each one having its own distinct aroma and flavour. These aromatic compounds provide many nutritional benefits and work like antioxidants in the body, helping defy the effects of ageing – mostly related to greying and loss of hair. So eat the variety which grows in the region you live.

PS: If you want a one-liner to remember the goodness of rice, here you go:

Rice is nice

7

Coconut
The Calmer

'Your children may not look after you in old age but the coconut tree will,' says a Tamil proverb. The kalpavriksha, the tree which will fulfil all your desires, emerged from the ocean along with the Kamadhenu (holy cow) during the churning of the ocean by the gods and the asuras. Needless to say, the coconut, also called shreefal, provides everything you need in life – it takes the saline water from the earth and turns it sweet, it gives you shade but just enough to not block the other crops from receiving their share of the sun, it will turn into a broom that will clean your house, you can make a sturdy home with its long leaves, it will burn as fuel, the hard shell of the coconut can turn into a vessel you can cook or even eat in, or you may simply eat the coconut in its many varieties – tender, ripe and dry. So basically, hard as a nut, at least in the Indian context, is a good thing.

Every morning in the filmi duniya of Mumbai, a coconut gets broken, its water is poured on the camera and other important equipment and every single person on the set bites into the fleshy coconut. The muhurat shot ka hero is the coconut. It is the hero because it will remove all obstacles and ward off every evil that stands in the way of the shoot – the permissions, the crowds or very simply the poker face of the ageing hero. Our culture draws this belief in the coconut as the vighnaharta, or remover of obstacles, from the fact that there is no other tree which takes salinity from the ground and turns it into nectar so sweet that you can actually shoot romantic scenes on Juhu beach with the hero–heroine drinking nariyal pani, two straws in one coconut.

On the outskirts of Mumbai is the Peshwa sea-fort town of Vasai, but even after the stupendous success of *Bajirao Mastani*, the only thing that interests the people of Mumbai in Vasai is not its history but its vegetables. The Vasaiwaali is the go-to bhajiwali and her vegetables are sold for a premium. The reason is that the bhaji grows in fields interspersed by coconut trees, which is known to enhance the fertility of the soil, keep it porous (mineral rich) and use up the salinity from the groundwater. This gives the bhaji from Vasai not just natural good looks and taste but its growers good money. Or, well, it used to. Till we became so health-conscious.

Our obsession with our health usually manifests itself in our tendency to scrutinize everything about our bodies from our sleep patterns to our blood sugar. And then comes the virtuous behaviour of eating idli but only with sambar or green chutney, and skipping the coconut. *Kyunki coconut mein cholesterol hai*, or so say the doctor, the dietician and even the good-looking celeb chef who sells olive oil. Or you are simply a fitness enthusiast who walks some 10,000 or whatever steps every day and one of the goals of your life is to avoid saturated fat. Or one day you were in the hospital with your granddad and the doc said no more coconut for you, it's not good for the heart and can cause diabetes, *aur aapne itne seriously le liya* that other than eating coconut cookies you have totally stayed off the nut.

The Miracle in Coconut

So anyways, *kya aap close-up karte hain, ya aap duniya se darte hai?* The truth, *deviyon aur sajjanon*, is that the coconut is divine. It has always been. The reason it is broken open at the beginning of not just a muhurat shot but basically at the start of any big project is that it gives the body endless physical stamina and the mind a sense of calm and reason. It's the effect of a magical group of essential fatty acids called medium-chain triglycerides (MCT), a fat similar to what's found in mother's milk.

MCT are much smaller than the large fatty acid molecules that you will find in, let's say, a Marie or a digestive biscuit. (It amazes me that processed fat biscuits are okayed by everyone and for everything; our desi coconut, ghee, etc., though are banned.) So these MCT get metabolized very differently in the human body compared to the other fats that we eat. They get preferentially used up for fuel, so you have more stamina or endurance. That's why MCT are also the preferred ergogenic aid (nutritional supplement) of endurance athletes, runners and cyclists alike.

MCT also have a role to play in myelination, that is, the forming of the myelin sheath around the nerves. You remember what that is, na? The white fatty layer around the nerves that helps in sending nerve impulses and also forms an electrical insulation around the nerves – axons, to sound very scientific. So myelination begins from the time you are in your mother's womb and will go on until adulthood – but here's the important thing: it helps in 'executive functioning', that is reasoning, planning and decision-making skills. Now isn't that exactly what you need your brain to do in tough situations like starting a project, getting married, having a baby, etc.? Now you know why it features everywhere in your dadi's plan of action?

Then there's the fact that just like ghee, fats from

coconut oil support the thyroid function and since thyroid is closely linked to brain function it improves our feeling of well-being. Add it all up, and the coconut is the ultimate calmer.

Fact vs Fiction

Fiction	Fact
Coconut is full of cholesterol	The MCT will help cut down the risk of cholesterol, and by the way, coconut is a plant food so it has no cholesterol. You need a liver to produce cholesterol. Reality check.
It's bad for the heart	Come on, coconut has such a good heart that it will never fall on anyone, and if it does, it's so rare that it will make news. The saturated fat from the coconut comes from a really special fatty acid called lauric acid. And lauric acid is not just good for the heart but also good for improving the body's fat-burning abilities.
Avoid if you are diabetic as it's high in fat	Exactly the reason why you should eat it, the fat. Addition of fat to meals reduces the glycaemic index and it's not just safe but recommended that diabetics eat meals that have a low glycaemic index.

Fiction	Fact
It's high calorie	The lauric acid and the other fatty acids in the coconut are known to improve satiety and thereby reduce the amount of calories consumed at any meal. That's why in India you garnish with coconut: it improves taste and prevents overeating.
Avoid if pregnant	Coconut has compounds that are known to kill pathogens and more specifically prevent yeast infections in the vaginal area. Getting sexually active or coming down with an infection? Grab a coconut.
Avoid if overweight	It's not the weight, dear, it's the body composition and more specifically it's your waist to hip ratio that decides whether you are at risk of developing obesity-related diseases. And hold your breath, the coconut is known to reduce the central adiposity, thereby reducing the risk of diseases. Want a slim waist? Don't look any further.

How to Have Coconut

Tender coconut water Better hydration than the colas and the sports drinks of the world. Improves renal function too. Woke up all hung over or with a splitting headache? Ditch the coffee and sip on tender coconut water. Nature's own refresher.

Tender coconut, commonly known as malai Scrape it from the insides of the tender coconut and chew on it slowly till it turns almost liquid and slips down your throat. Great to build the health of your intestines; especially useful for chronic constipation, IBS, ulcerative colitis and Crohn's disease.

Ripe and fleshy coconut From coping with heartbreak, forgiving backstabbers, improving satiety to better fat-burning or simply learning to eat the right amount, the coconut will help you with everything. Really trying to knock off the need to smoke or drown in a coffee post-lunch? Just garnish your food with coconut. And like the coastal folk do, cook your curries in coconut. Rice and fish or veg curry in coconut is a strong contender for the ultimate heart-healthy meal. But then it's too yummy and we unfortunately put yucky and healthy in the same bracket.

Dry coconut Often mixed with other seeds like

alshi (flax), til (sesame), peanuts, etc., depending on the region you come from, it makes for a great chutney and is a part of the laddoos that are specially recommended during and post-pregnancy. The laddoos give you the fat-burning and satiety-improving benefits of MCT and are also a way of providing them in concentrated doses to help little babies get going with the myelination and even prevent post-partum depression in young mothers.

Coconut oil The new virgin on the oil shelves of the West, coconut oil is among the latest heart health discoveries for the West. Our Malayali brethren, on the other hand, were urged, almost forced, to get off it to protect their hearts. Typically, in Kerala, the grandparents are still cooking in coconut oil, the parents are using vegetable oils and the young kids are on olive oil. No prizes for guessing who has the strongest heart of them all. From deep-frying banana chips to lending a distinct flavour to the aviyal or as a tadka on the pachhadi, coconut oil enriches not just our meals but also our scalp with lustrous, thick and dandruff-free hair.

8

Aliv
The Beauty Pill

'F***!' exclaimed Vanshika, as she got up from her chair and walked to the window. 'You know what I have done, right?' she said, staring out of the window. 'I have flushed down every one of those laddoos that my dadi saas sent up to my room, post-pregnancy. That's forty-five of them. Two minutes' silence for bitches like me.' She turned towards me, face filled with rage. I thought she was going to knock me down but then she burst into tears and the rest, as they say, is history.

She is not alone. Hordes of Indian women can't bear the post-pregnancy fussing of MIL and MM (monster moms) over their food. They are desperate to get back in shape post-pregnancy and feel that everything these older ladies offer is 'fattening'. There's ghee, coconut and more ghee in the halwa, in the laddoo, even in their glass of milk.

By now you no longer need convincing about the miracles of ghee and coconut and how these are actually super-fat-burning and calming agents for the body. What is really sad is that in our quest to avoid ghee and coconut, we have avoided some brilliant seeds that they are mixed with and turned into laddoos. No, I am not talking about fenugreek, or methi seeds, which has found acceptance here now that the West has accepted it as a lactation enhancer; I am talking about the lesser-known scarlet-coloured aliv seeds, also called halim or garden cress.

Aliv seeds, and more specifically their laddoos, have always been an integral part of India's strictly followed code of what women must and must not eat post-pregnancy. Ayurveda recognizes aliv as an important part of the post-partum diet. Even the Prophet himself is said to have recommended it to his followers. It grows easily in small pots and even in the wild by lakes and ponds. Indian tribals collect these from the forest and feed them to infants or young mommies in the village.

The Miracle in Aliv

Aliv is full of so many miracles that sometimes it strikes me as a tragedy that its benefits are not fully known or celebrated. Traditionally, grandmas would soak these seeds in coconut water and then cook them with grated coconut, ghee and jaggery and roll them into bright red laddoos. These laddoos are the ultimate power foods. Aliv is a rich source of essential fatty acids like linoleic and arachidic, and when it is mixed with coconut and ghee you get the perfect ratio of omega 3, 6, 9. The laddoos keep the postpartum blues away and also allow you to assimilate all the micronutrients hidden in the aliv, like folic acid and minerals like iron and calcium.

Post-pregnancy, a woman tackles many changes not just in her body but also in her hair. Ya, you heard that right. Loss of hair is among the most common issues that a woman faces when she's in a hormonal flux – the lactation period and menopause being classic examples. This was one reason Vanshika had her meltdown that day. She wanted me to help her with her hair loss and I had suggested an aliv laddoo a day as a mid-meal. The phytonutrients, iron and amino acids in garden cress help prevent the oxidative stresses that lead to hair loss, thinning, split ends, etc., and help retain both the density and lustre of the hair.

And it's not just hair. Aliv could well be our most well-guarded beauty secret because along with vitamins A and E it has this nutrient called sulforaphane, which provides the skin with an even tone, rids it of patches and naturally brightens the skin. Sounds like nature's own Fair and Lovely, doesn't it? Little wonder then that Ayurveda chooses to put it high on its list of post-partum food – good hair and good skin make any girl feel better about herself.

Aliv has one more trick up its potent sleeve. In Africa, the seeds are not just regarded as a post-partum essential but as a natural aphrodisiac because it has properties that mimic estrogen and energy-giving minerals. In India, pregnancy is considered a rebirth for women, and it's almost as if aliv makes you come alive both sexually and aesthetically all over again.

PCOD, or polycystic ovarian disease

The current epidemic that afflicts the superwomen of India is PCOD. One that gives you too much testosterone, too little hair on the scalp and too many on the face. The acne and pimples don't seem to disappear and the periods are forever playing hide-and-seek. You have to cope with the burden of being overweight too. And then we make the same mistakes that new mothers make. Shun everything that's considered fattening – the ghee mostly– and thus you miss out on all the laddoos that get made at home (like aliv) that could provide your body with natural good looks, regulate your periods, reduce your bloating and help you get rid of those bald patches.

Anyways, for all the men reading this and wondering *mera kya*, don't worry, aliv works like an aphrodisiac for both men and women. Now surely you wouldn't mind eating aliv to get into the mood, especially post-childbirth.

How to Eat Aliv

Aliv sprouts One way to eat garden cress if you want it for skin-brightening purposes – is to turn it into a chutney; in high-end restaurants (where it is the latest trend), the sprouts are added to soups.

Aliv greens The baby greens that you see everywhere these days. On the side of that egg dish that you ordered in London, on top of the pizza when it's gourmet or simply as a garnish on your sandwiches. The West is loving the way it looks and the multiple health benefits it has. Give it the right PR and it could well be the next big hot trend in India.

Aliv seeds This is the comfort zone. This is how India has been eating them. Soak them overnight and turn them into laddoos or kheer or simply add a teaspoon to milk. From strength to vigour, from good looks to fertility, from curing anaemia and a weak stomach, this one is good for all ages, all genders, all classes.

Aliv oil Very niche use, smells similar to mustard oil. So you could use it as seasoning and even for external application, especially on cracked lips.

Special Note: Aliv and Cancer

It was in 2003 that for the first time I had a client sign up for a diet because she was fighting breast cancer. The number steadily rose but until 2007 it was still in single digits. And now every month my team or I are working with a new client with breast cancer. 'The thing is that they come from all kinds of backgrounds and age groups,' I mentioned to a Delhi oncologist over a casual conversation over coffee. 'The only similarity that I can see is that most, if not all, of them have crash-dieted post-pregnancy, especially after the second one.' The oncologist, only busy with his coffee till now, looked up and said to me, 'It's interesting you say that. And it is totally possible because the body is in such a hormonal flux, and if you cut down drastically on calories, immunity drops and then it could get to you. You need protective fats and micronutrient-rich meals because at any point cancer cells are present in the body, but we are all depending on the body's ability to regress them.'

This is where aliv comes into the picture. It is a rich source of something called BITC, or benzyl isothiocyanate. Now this is almost like a wonder drug because studies have proved that it has strong properties that work as a powerful deterrent to cancer cells. This also makes it a chemo protective agent, one that protects healthy cells from the toxic effect of anti-cancer drugs.

Aliv, with its estrogenic properties, rich micronutrients and cancer-protecting abilities, is just everything that you need to lead a good, healthy life. It's the chhota bomb with the bada effect on your health and well-being.

9

Jackfruit
The Fertility Booster

Every year at least one jackfruit of mine gets stolen. It both annoys and amuses me. The jackfruit is officially India's largest fruit, the largest fruit that any tree can ever bear. It is seriously heavy and you need two hands and sometimes even four to pick up a single fruit with some villages down south claiming that their jackfruit is as heavy as 70 kilos. Whatever the veracity of that claim, a jackfruit weighing 10 to 15 kilos is really, really regular.

In the Konkan region, of which the jackfruit is a native, the world can be divided into mango and jackfruit lovers. I belong to the latter. With thorns on the outside and sweetness on the inside, the jackfruit imitates its native people, always ready with a few cuss words but with a heart of gold – just like the sunshine-coloured, carotene and the anthocyanin-rich jackfruit, bulbs which sit together around the fibrous stem. Though the jackfruit is a native of the Western Ghats, it grows well in all tropical regions of India, especially down south, and even up north, where it is called kathal.

Among the first migrants to Mumbai were people from Konkan. But the thing about us folks from Konkan is that, even three generations later, we will make at least one yearly trip to Konkan. And mostly we will all make it around the phanas or jackfruit time and bring it back to Mumbai in the trunk of a bus, and that's where it gets stolen from. But we know that everyone wants a piece of jackfruit, so we bring at least two to account for one being stolen. The one that you are left with is large enough to feed the entire mohalla.

A girl who learns to cut open a jackfruit can wade smoothly through life. She must learn where to apply pressure, when to go hard, how to go soft but still be steady and, most important, she should know where to make the cut. Life-saving skills, if you ask me. One of my grandfathers taught me how to cut open a jackfruit and the other one, a coconut. The coconut is broken assuming the badhakon posture and the jackfruit, upavishta konasana. Both the postures and the fruit are critical for reproductive health, preventing PMS and acne, especially the acne around the chin and on the forehead. I can peel both from the outer covering and ideally this should go in my CV because it basically means that I can rise to any occasion, break open the hardest exterior and make a smooth entry into the deep, inner, sweet flesh. Fruitgasm anybody? It sure is a skill that has helped me with my work – the hardest of exteriors doesn't bother me, I know that all it takes is knife skills;)

We no longer value these skills or the taste of the jackfruit or its multiple uses and this has landed the jackfruit in the NUS list of the UNFAO. And that's because it is unfortunately considered a poor man's fruit in its native country. In addition, the very virtue of jackfruit, its heady sweetness, has won it the reputation of being a fattening or a sugary fruit.

We would rather talk of blueberries and kiwi or say things like an apple a day...for health and weight loss. There is more prestige associated in taking exotic fruits than native ones.

Bangladesh though regards the jackfruit as its national fruit. That apart, our local, native fruit is now being grown by California farmers and is being targeted at the health- and environment-conscious crowds on the West Coast. It's considered the food of the future, a vegan, gluten-free protein alternative to meat. As a fruit rich in phenolic compounds and antioxidants. As a high-fibre flour with laxative properties that can cure the most constipated of systems. All in all, the usual story – introduce a novel food item from Asia or Africa, adapt it to western taste and peg it on health and wellness and watch it turn red-hot.

The Running Grandfather

The nariyal pani wala outside my office in Mumbai is a native of Kerala, his dada is a 94-year-old, a five time namazi. But he goes to the mosque for every namaz, doesn't just spread the mat, take of his shoes and pray wherever he is. The dada has just been detected with cancer, but he has a good doctor who has told the family that no treatment is needed, just keep a watch over him. So the grandsons now want to keep him home and don't let him go to the mosque. The grandfather has lived 94 years and is in good health (clinical aspect aside), and all his life he has eaten jackfruit in all its forms – raw, ripe, seeds, fried and even rolled it into a chapatti. So he slips out and runs (actually runs) to the mosque, the grandsons run after him, the whole village has a good laugh and all is well with their world.

The drought-resistant jackfruit will bear multiple fruits every year and, like its native cousin coconut, can be used in many versatile ways. The veena, the musical instrument the goddess Saraswati carries and which is played at dhrupad concerts, is made from the wood of the jackfruit. The value of both the dhrupad and the veena is disappearing from our homes and is beginning to find appreciation in the West. The wood of the jackfruit also lends itself to the tala of the mridangam and many other musical instruments. The robes that monks in South East Asia wear use a dye that comes from the jackfruit tree.

The Magic Ingredient

Bala Ganapati, the child form of Ganesha, who bestows youth, exuberance and enthusiasm on all who worship him, carries a jackfruit in his hand for a reason. It's a fruit that can help improve your insulin sensitivity. Ageing is a natural phenomenon, but loss of energy and enthusiasm is not. That's caused by insulin resistance, a condition where your cells don't receive the nourishment that's their due, causing them to shrink and eventually wither away.

The enthusiasm for jackfruit in the health food segment stems, among many other reasons, from its ability to improve insulin sensitivity associated with sustainable weight loss and regulation of blood sugars. This special quality of the jackfruit may be due to a number of factors – the insulin-mimicking from its minerals, the improved metabolism from its vitamins, the slow release of blood sugars from its fibres or simply from the joyful state of mind that the jackfruit can put you in. Insulin resistance happens to be the key reason for irregular periods and ovulation, and can lead to infertility. And this is why this overlooked fruit may be your secret weapon to getting pregnant.

Fact vs Fiction

Fiction	Fact
It's fattening	Sweetness is a virtue when it exists naturally and is not made in some industrial unit. Low on fat and rich in fibre, the jackfruit will help reduce cholesterol levels. Won't make you fat but fit.

Fiction	Fact
It's smelly	Of course, it has a distinct fragrance. You can smell it from a distance and it is exactly these volatile phenolic compounds that give it antioxidant properties. Can help reduce menopausal pigmentation too.
It's not hygienic	That depends on how you define hygiene. With a shell that covers it completely, it is almost impossible for it to spoil, but it is perishable. So learn when to pick them off the tree, bring them home, sit around as a family to peel it. It's more fun than sharing a glass of champagne or watching TV or a film together.
It's for the poor	It's highly perishable so you don't really see it in rich people's stores. It won't survive their logistical, delivery-chain journey. Dehydrated and packaged ones are slowly making their way to the Indian markets but most of it is still exported. Anything but the poor man's fruit, it's the new super-fruit on the weight-loss circuit.

How to Eat It

There are multiple ways you can use the jackfruit. Here are some:

Leaves Idlis and dosas are wrapped in jackfruit leaves in some regions. The phytonutrients enhance the flavour of the idli–dosa and the minerals help boost your immune system.

Raw jackfruit Forget all the talk of beef being the poor man's protein source; raw jackfruit is the real deal: India's very own mock-meat even before it became fashionable to mock meat or go vegan. Phanas or kathal sabzi is a delicacy in every region of India. It is a storehouse of nutrients and especially good for fighting bloating and restoring hormonal balance. Also used to make pure veg biryanis where the raw jackfruit takes on the delicious flavours and aromas of the original meat biryani.

Ripe jackfruit There are mainly two varieties of jackfruit, the one with hard bulbs called kapa and the slimy one called barka. Both have their own fan base. I belong to the kapa team. There is no fruit sweeter or more regal-looking than jackfruit bulbs. A storehouse of antioxidants that can fight carcinogens and with fibres that maintain a diverse ecosystem of gut-friendly bacteria, the jackfruit is like the anti-ageing insurance that you cannot afford to miss on. It's great for maintaining the health of the colon and gall bladder too.

Jackfruit seeds When you eat the fruit, save the seeds and sun-dry them. Later you can boil or roast them or make atta out of them. Rich in vitamin B, they possess an enviable amino acid profile. A popular way to eat them is like an usal or a dal and have it with rice, garnished with coconut. There isn't a more exotic way to get a complete meal than this. The UN declared 2016 as the year of pulses essentially to bring these kind of lost and forgotten seeds back in focus. Do your bit, eat the jackfruit seed this year. And don't forget this – if you have been on too many diets and troubled all your organs, this is what you need to heal.

Chips, papad and flattened sweet rotis At various stages the jackfruit can be turned into chips that you have with coffee, papad to have with dahi rice, and sweet rotis to have like a mid-afternoon snack. Each one has a distinct flavour, unique nutritional values and is delicious to taste. *Sab kuch hai, bas marketing ki kami hai;)*

Thorny outer shell This would go to the cattle at home because it improves the quality of milk that cows produce, and it is especially given to nursing or pregnant cows. The only thing that you have got to be careful about is the beam that runs across the fruit, which needs to be discarded. The beam can be used as manure but not as food for cattle as it could mess with their heads and even lead to madness.

10

Sugar
The Anti-Ageing Secret

The Omnipresent Sugar Cane

When King Siddhartha opened his eyes after the seventh week of his enlightenment, sugar cane was the first food he ate. The first Jain teerthankara, Rishabadeva, broke his year-long fast with sugar cane juice. Jainism, like Buddhism, has the same sweet teaching of ahimsa.

After Chaturmasa, four months of deep sleep, Lord Vishnu wakes up enlightened and rejuvenated and marries Tulsi, a native plant celebrated for its many therapeutic properties. Sugar cane is the main offering at the wedding, and it marks the beginning of the harvest of sugar cane, one of India's oldest crops. Farmers celebrate this by offering five stalks of sugar cane, one each to a Brahmin, blacksmith, washerman, barber and water-woman, and one they keep for themselves. The gesture has its origins in Advaita, a school of philosophy in Hinduism that preaches oneness. Though outwardly we are all different, performing different tasks in society, at the core we are all the same. Just like sugar cane, each stalk looks different but crush it or pound it and you get the same sugar, same sweetness.

Tripurasundari, the tantric goddess who signifies eternal youth and beauty, carries sugar cane in one of her four arms, signifying that bliss, beauty and sweetness are the basis of all existence. It's worth remembering for all of us who want to quit sugar to become more beautiful that the goddess who signifies not just beauty but also youth and innocence is a believer of sugar. And she is saying that it's not your size that can make you beautiful but what shines through your body.

Tripurasundari, the Buddha and Vishnu evoke the same subtle message in these stories – there is harmony in diversity. This harmony is achieved when you reach the essence, the essence is found when the outer layer is discarded and so the metaphor of sugar cane all the time. Pundaraka (another name for sugar cane; pundra = to crush or turn into powder) is crushed to reveal the same colourless, crystalline sugar, the same sweetness.

History of Sugar – Part 1

Sugar Goes from India to the Rest of the World

Shakkara, Sanskrit for sugar, is mentioned in the Rig Veda, Charaka Samhita and Sushruta Samhita and has been in use as medicine and food and for ritualistic purposes in India since time immemorial. It is one of the panchamrits, the five nectars of life. There are references to crystalline sugar from the Gupta period (320–550 CE) and even earlier to sugar mills in Buddhist texts.

Ancient India had perfected the art of refining sugar from sugar cane and there were specific names for every grade of refining. Every by-product of refining from the concentrated syrup to the purest, colourless, crystalline molecules of sugar had a specific use and also applications in medicine according to the ancient texts. Charaka used sugar to cure digestion-related ailments, improve complexion and even increase sperm production. The *Arthashastra* describes how sugar can be used to increase the strength and vigour of elephants. And the Mahabharata mentions using a sugar cane by-product with spices to make a fragrant wine.

China documents at least two missions that came to India to learn the art of refining sugar after Buddhism took its teaching and sugar cane to China. Ibn Battuta, the Arabic traveller, mentions having a sugary drink called sherbet in Delhi and Alexander's army described the use of a sweet salt in milk – someone had a nice kheer I am guessing.

So if you come from this land and legacy and consider that sugar is white poison then it's really a shame, unless of course you are talking about colonization. One of the main drivers of the colonization of our country was the trade of sugar along with spices. It also led in part to slavery in

Africa and indentured labour in West Indies. I am
no history professor or intellectual but you look at
how every colonized nation is now a middle- or
low-income country, how it has so much political
instability. And I think one of the reasons it is like
this is that colonies that used sugar cane to enslave
us, colonize us, used sugar cane only for economic
benefits and our differences to divide and rule.

If the West is paranoid about sugar, damn good,
they ought to be. They never learned that inner
harmony and not economy was the message of sugar
cane. If you cause instability on the very land that
you make your wealth from, then karma has got a
way to get you, man.

A Short History of the Parsis

Long ago a group of people from Persia came
seeking refuge to the coast of Sajjan in Gujarat.
Jadi Rana, the king of Sajjan, politely declined

their request by showing them a vessel full to the brim with milk, to signify that the kingdom was already full and couldn't accept any more people. The leader of the group then stepped forward and added sugar to the milk to signify that his people would live on his land, like sugar in milk. Without changing its colour, its odour or its characteristics but only by lending the sweetness they had. India is now home to this group and, true to the word of their leader, the Parsis have only enhanced India.

History of Sugar – Part 2

Sugar Fear Comes from the West to India

In my summer school in Potsdam, Germany, I learned that the West changed the way they were eating following the two world wars. As nations became more industrialized and women stepped out to work, there was less time to cook and ready-to-eat meals and eating out became the norm. The food business, like any other business, is about the bottom line and the best way to improve that is to get ingredients and use technology that will make you feel that you are still eating food but unlike real food these will not have the problems of perishability and loss of taste with time, and who cares about the loss of nutrients. Sugar made way for beet sugar and HFCS, or high fructose corn syrup. They were easy to procure, easy to handle and, most important, cheaper.

A lot of the press, reports and research that you read about the evils of sugar include information about beet sugar and HFCS (see box below for more on these). **The problem here is that the food model of Western society is being passed off as the face of science.**

With nutrition transition we started eating more packaged and processed food, a westernization of lifestyle basically. With it we are consuming more added sugars like HFCS. And while in Europe it took several decades for this change to occur, in countries like ours it's happening in just one generation. You eat cereal milk for breakfast and your cousin, just ten years older, can't bear the thought of starting her day with a cold, sugary breakfast. She wants something hot and salty not sweet and cold. The world is changing the way it is eating and we are eating more like each other than unlike each other. More packaged cereals, more juices, more soda, more cupcakes, everything more than ever.

Beet Sugar and HFCS

Beet sugar came into existence during the Napoleonic wars. Napoleon came out with policies that almost forced farmers to grow beet sugar in France. From there it made its journey into the rest of Europe and even the US, where Japanese Americans displaced during the Second World War were used as labour to grow the beet sugar.

When you go abroad and add your regular one sachet of sugar to your coffee, it doesn't seem quite enough. The reason is that what you get as sugar in the West is mostly beet sugar and for our palettes that are used to sugar from sugar cane, it doesn't quite do it. To make this more complex, a lot of the beet sugar is derived from the GMO variety of beet plants. And in the US you don't have to say where the sugar is coming from, beet or sugar cane, it's just simply labelled sugar. There is no separate labelling for GMO also. Last year in Miami, I walked into a coffee store and stopped at the sugar counter and among at least five different types of sugars and sweeteners found a sachet of 'cane sugar'. So the latest thing in the West is that sugar is bad and all but cane sugar is natural and non-GM.

By the way, Rishabadeva wouldn't have juice that came from beet because Jainism doesn't eat root veggies like beet. So for us Indians, sucrose is not just sucrose, the source matters, incredible India and all.

HFCS or iso-glucose is a chemically derived form of sugar that comes from corn, the American corn that you also get at stalls when you go to the movies. Because the US has hefty taxes on sugar but big subsidies for corn, it's much cheaper and easier to use HFCS in every packaged food item as a sweetening agent. The corn industry has tried to pass this sugar as natural but thankfully it isn't legal yet to call it natural sugar. From packaged cereals to juices to colas, most packaged food and drink products have this type of sugar.

HFCS is the form of sugar that is most linked to metabolic disorders like obesity and diabetes. Soft drink companies have been using HFCS in colas in the US since 1984 but in Mexico they use sugar. So you will find the dardi Mexicans going to the local Mexican grocery store to get their cola. During the Passover festival of Jews, companies sell colas with sugar as HFCS is not considered kosher. Interesting, na? The point is that apart from the common quality of sweetness, real sugar from cane is completely different from HFCS. Thinking that HFCS is sugar is like thinking domestic violence is like love.

Giving Up on Cane

Even as I write this, scientists in the West are beginning to study what they call cane sugar and its benefits for the body. So expect to hear more of the good stuff and at least some distinction between different kinds of sugar. In the meanwhile, we are turning sugar sceptics and swallowing the Western attack against sugar wholesale.

How We Once Ate Sugar	How We Eat It Now
Culturally acceptable and recommended for centuries Sugar cane derivatives	Globalization happens. Westernization pushes its way in as a more intelligent, hygienic, cooler choice. Mostly, if not every time, commercial and low-grade beet or corn sugar is used. If you have Indian DNA you have not been exposed to this for more than 10, max 20, years.
Cow milk, diluted cow milk and halwas for infants and toddlers	Infant formulas almost from birth High in sugars and no source specified
Kesar, dry fruit or gulkand/chyawanprash in milk for school kids	Powders with high amount of industrialized sugar parading around as protein-rich, iron-rich, vitamin-D-rich additions to milk for brain and growth, etc.

How We Once Ate Sugar	How We Eat It Now
Easy, quick, nutrient-rich homemade meals: sheera and halwa, dalia, poha, upma, idli, dosa, paratha	Ready-to-eat cereals with HFCS. The joke is that they are for weight loss. Bharat Dabholkar, the big ad guy, told an audience on a panel he was sharing with me that an MNC making cereals pumped in crores for advertising in India and doesn't care about profits for the first 10 years. They just want to project their cereal as a healthier alternative to local breakfast options.
Chai or coffee with its share of sugar Eaten with a handful of peanuts or makhana at chai time	Use sweetener for chai and coffee or simply have it without sugar but always with a Marie biscuit or a cookie. Needless to say, both have added sugar of the exact variety that you should be avoiding.
Fresh fruit or homemade sherbets	Canned juices, flavoured powders, colas

How We Once Ate Sugar	How We Eat It Now
Homemade laddoos made according to the season used as mid-meal snacks	Designer shops offering cupcakes at every nook and corner. Of course they also serve cookies and you can even have cookie milkshakes.
Homemade shrikhand made with curd which was hung overnight	Greek yogurt, fruit yogurt, ice creams, etc.
Homemade seasonal delicacies like halwa, sheera, laddoos, barfis, mixture of sugar cane and its derivatives, with nutritious local grains and pulses and dry fruit and ghee – minerals that mimic insulin, fibre that releases blood sugar slowly, ghee that reduces the glycaemic index of food, vitamins that fight free radical damage	Even Diwali hampers now have chocolates, Ganapati modaks are made of chocolates and baby arrivals announced with brownies, cookies and cupcakes. Low-grade sugar or sweeteners, with flours devoid of fibre, cocoa from another continent, preservatives, additives, colouring agents, trans-fat or low-grade-fat alternatives. Since the 1970s, India's sugar consumption has tripled.

Fructose

The naturally existing fruit sugar is best enjoyed when a fruit is eaten as a whole and not when it is juiced. Juice delivers a whole lot of fructose at one shot and evolution has not taught our bodies to cope with it. A lot of the negative reports about sugar also include fructose. There are even reports to show that fructose can be more harmful than glucose. You don't need to worry about these technicalities if you like to chew your fruit. But if you are choosing a fruit juice over a sherbet or having a cold pressed juice for its supposedly health benefits, you are putting your body at risk.

Science Keeps Changing Its Mind

The problem with nutrition science is that it keeps changing its mind. In 1999, fat was the major villain, sugar was okay. By 2015, we had swung around to arguing that fat was not responsible for obesity and obesity-related diseases, it was sugar. After summer school, I attended the FENS conference (nutrition societies from all across Europe participate in it) in Berlin and at one of the talks an economics professor joked that in nutrition exams the question was always the same but the answers changed every year. Basically he was saying that nutrition science is cuckoo science. I mean look at us, is cholesterol bad? Yes, in 2014. Come 2015, no, the US FDA says it's 'an essential nutrient that is no longer a concern for overconsumption'. The economics professor further emphasized that food should be a multidisciplinary study, one that includes politics, history, sociology, nutrition and economics.

Every five years when big countries review their nutrition guidelines, your villain until yesterday becomes your fat-loss aid and vice versa. Guidelines for sugar have been changing too and dramatically at that. When I passed out of school in 1999 there was no official upper limit for consumption of sugar. Then in 2002 WHO said we had to cut down sugar to 10 per cent of our total calorie intake and in 2015 the American Heart Association made a further distinction, reducing sugar use to 5 per cent of daily calories from 'added sugars', that is, excluding fruits and dairy.

Evidence-Based Latest Sugar Guidelines

Health Body	Guidelines	In Tsp (Men–Women)
WHO	10 per cent of daily calorie intake	17.5–12.5
	5 per cent of additional benefits	9–6
UK NHS	5 per cent of daily calorie intake	9–6
USFDA	10 per cent of daily calorie intake	17.5–12.5
American Heart Association	5 per cent of daily calorie intake	9–6

Now when you come from India where your grandma gets upset when you talk about, not to mention count, how many rotis or pooris you have eaten, how do you account for daily calorie consumption, much less requirement? And if you do go by some calorie count that's required by adults, you make the mistake that the eco prof warns against: of not accounting for cultural, genetic, environmental differences and of failing to understand the relevance of granny's advice and taking part in being the cuckoo of the science.

When your grandma put granules of sugar on your palm when you left her home every summer vacation to return to yours and to school life, what exactly was she thinking? Was she thinking you have been a pain in my ass, may these granules of sugar make you fat, diabetic and dull so that you don't return here for your next vacation? Or is she thinking, hold infinity in the palm of your hand, eternity in your hour, like Blake wrote? Like she was taught by her grandma who learned the tantric wisdom of Tripurasundari or from Buddhism or simply from the almost revolutionary abhangas that were written for Vitthala with generous metaphors of sugar cane. Maybe she's already in tune with the current buzzword, sustainability. And all that she stands to gain is your charming company so that she may teach you by leading an exemplary life where she doesn't fear food, much less sugar.

Sugar Cane's Magic Properties

Sugar cane puts your body in the positive nitrogen balance. That is a state where the body is not sacrificing muscle to meet its energy demands and it could well be the reason why its juice has been used to break fasts right from the Buddha's time. Loss of muscle, especially the type that comes with being constantly on a weight-loss spree, is actually one of the factors that ages the body. Believe it or not, sugar cane provides fibre, minerals and even vitamin B, all of which help the body keep the digestive system strong; and you do know that with age digestion loses its power, don't you? When you make a juice out of it, with the roller blades moving smoothly and slowly on every cane, you actually manage to retain most of the nutrients, but you have to drink it on the spot for the benefits. It's antioxidant-rich so it cannot be stored.

Sugar cane and all its derivatives also have

glycolic acid (in varying amounts), the same AHA (alpha hydroxy acid) that you find written in bold on cosmetic products. From the high streets of New York to the posh shops at international airports, everyone's talking about sugar in their lip balm, body scrubs and even face packs. It helps prevent skin damage of all kinds, from tanning to freckles to wrinkles. That's such a sweet anti-ageing secret to have.

Fact vs Fiction

Fiction	Fact
Avoid if diabetic	Meta studies show no conclusive link between consumption of sugar and occurrence of diabetes. But increase in consumption of processed foods like biscuits, breads, colas, ice creams is positively associated with risk of diabetes and heart disease.
	Chronic diabetics are in fact often asked to keep sugar on them, to prevent hypoglycaemia. Can't be a bigger testimony than that to sugar's blood-sugar-regulating properties.

Fiction	Fact
	Also note that India and China have among the lowest per capita consumption of sugar in the world. So it's not the sugar which is the main cause behind diabetes, it's the lifestyle. For example, TV viewing is linked to inactivity, irregular mealtimes and disturbed sleep, all precursors of insulin resistance.

If you keep up with your native, regional eating habits, even with the halwa or laddoo, 2–3 cups of chai, you won't even reach 4–5 tsp per day, that's less than the prescribed guidelines. And that too of sugar, not HFCS. |
| Avoid if you want to lose weight | Obesity is linked with processed food and sedentary lifestyle. Eating a cereal for its promise of weight loss over poha, upma, paratha, idli, dalia? The poor quality sugar from weight-loss products will add to your weight, not sugar from daily traditional diets. |
| Better to use low- or no-calorie sweeteners | Sweeteners, however low in calories or endorsed by celebrities, have no health benefits whatsoever. First, the brain has neurons or plain smartness to detect |

Fiction	Fact
	that you are cheating it, so you will crave and consume more calories than you have saved. Second, reported side effects are anywhere from dull thyroid, memory loss to cancer.
How about stevia, it's natural	Boss, sugar cane is not natural, kya? How disconnected we are with the soil and connected with the Wi-Fi. We know that stevia is a plant from the South Americas but don't know that sugar cane is a plant which could be growing just about 30 kilometres from our physical location and its relevance in our culture. Anyways, in the early 1990s the US had banned stevia because its toxicology report said it was unsafe for consumption and was a carcinogenic and then in 2008 accepted it to sweeten colas.
Will just add jaggery instead of sugar because it's healthier	Everything that comes from the sugar cane plant is healthy but has its own distinct effect on the human body. Jaggery adds to the warmth of the body and is consumed as winter food along with ghee. It also takes away sharp odours from cooking. Sugar on

Fiction	Fact
	the other hand is a coolant, to be used in summers even as a digestive aid. It enhances flavours in cooking. In chai or coffee if you used jaggery instead of sugar, it would make it even hotter for the body and take away their distinct aromas.
Honey is better than sugar	It is sweet but molecularly different from sugar. So use it where appropriate to enhance certain dishes, to mix Ayurvedic medicines with or to ease a sore throat. It is, however, not an alternative or replacement for sugar cane and its many derivatives.
Sugar causes cavities	If you chew on a gum with a sugar substitute or eat sugar-substituted chocolates, yogurts and ice creams, it's going to do nothing good for your oral health. Chocolates, juices, ice creams, colas and sodas are just bad for oral health and there is no way around that. Chewing on sugar cane and spitting out its fibre (in the right place), however, is a great way of keeping good oral health. In fact, if you can't bite off a sugar cane, it's time to visit

Fiction	Fact
	a dentist. Eating a homemade laddoo, made with natural fibre and antioxidant-rich ingredients like rava, besan, ragi, etc., is good for oral health. And that's because after eating a homemade ladoo or halwa, nothing sticks in the gap of your teeth, and left to rot.
But why have sugar at all, our body converts all food to glucose anyways	That sounds like now that I am married I can get out of shape or something as random as that. Everything will get broken down to glucose but it has its own specific pathways. Depending on how, when, with what and with whom you eat it, the exact same food will respond differently in your body. Sugar is the sweetest of all foods, and it will get broken down to glucose too but that shouldn't be held against it. Also remember that sugar is a good delivery agent, makes it easy for your body to assimilate nutrients and bioactive compounds. Homeopathy uses sugar pills to deliver the medicine. So your body can use sugar and you can abuse it. There's a fine line there.

How to Have Sugar

Sugar Cane

1. Stalks of sugar cane are chewed across India during the winters. In western Maharashtra, there's a celebration of the winter produce called the *hoorda* party. On the menu is hoorda (tender jowar), sugar cane, bor (jujube), each one with its own unique therapeutic property but the underlying one is that of improved hormonal balance leading to enhanced fertility levels. You could think of this as our native version of Valentine's Day. But the chances of your knowing about pumpkin carving for Halloween are higher than of your knowing about the native hoorda party or its version in your region.

2. Sugar cane is used in Ayurvedic medicine for a deep cleanse and detox. That's one reason why this is what you chew on or drink as medicine for jaundice. It actually helps in recovery and rejuvenation of the liver.

3. Cold pressed sugar cane juice (yeah! native technique of crushing stalks together beat the cold press trend by centuries) is a well-known digestive aid.

Kakvi or Molasses before Turning into Jaggery

1. A semi-liquid state, dark in colour and with the consistency of honey, often eaten with chapattis as a complete meal.
2. Rich in minerals, can fight off the free radical effect of ageing on organs.
3. It's a native version of an 'alkaline' diet, promotes a healthier, more diverse ecosystem of gut-friendly bacteria
4. Folk medicine for kidney stones.

Jaggery or Gud

1. Solid state, dark to light brown in colour, celebrated for its ability to give warmth to the body.
2. Is a compulsory accompaniment to bajra rotis and is mixed with ghee to assimilate the

nutrients from bajra better.

3. Used as a mouth freshener after meals, can remove the odour that comes after eating raw onions and garlic.

4. Ayurvedic medicine for improving haemoglobin levels and part of traditional pregnancy diets.

5. Effectively prevents cold, cough and flu.

Sugar

1. Comes in various forms – big chunks called khadi sakhar, small tiny cubes called mishri and the commonly found granulated sugar.

2. Celebrated for its role as a catalyst, driving energy and nutrients into the cell membranes of the body, making metabolism itself possible.

3. Khadi sakhar is traditionally used by classical artists to hold at the back of their jaws while doing their riyaz. Known to make the vocal chords or the voicebox more flexible, breathing deeper and voice sweeter.

4. Also used in traditional Ayurvedic medicines, mixed with herbs and roots. Makes delivery and assimilation of bioactive molecules in the body easier.

5. Mishri mixed with clove is used for fighting tooth decay and even motion sickness.

6. Mishri mixed with spices is also used as an effective aid against sinus and headaches.

7. Granulated sugar or shakar is one of the five panchamrits. A pinch added to sabzis or dals, it is often the secret ingredient in every chef's recipe.

8. Known as a digestive aid, it is used in many traditional sherbets to improve hydration status, accelerate recovery and reduce acidity in the body.

9. Mixed in traditional laddoos and halwas along with mineral-rich grains, essential fatty-acid–rich nuts and ghee, it makes for a versatile ingredient that doesn't take away from the therapeutic properties of what it is mixed with.

10. It is Passed around and celebrated on days or moments that are worth remembering because it's a brain fuel too. That's how you have the *mooh meetha kar lo* system.

11. Often mixed with ghee so that rise in blood sugars is slower, steadier, leading to long-lasting effects of energy and well-being.

12. Mixed with dahi, used as an aid to build a healthier gut ecosystem. Often eaten during exams and long travels, as stressful environments come in the way of healthy gut bacteria.

13. Mixed with milk, haldi and kesar as an immunity booster and as an aid to prevent signs of ageing on the skin.

Appendix: Regional Names of Aliv, Ambadi and Kokum

Aliv*

Allibija, alavibija (Kannada)
Asali (Malayalam)
Asaliya (Gujarati)
Adiyalu, adeli (Telugu)
Ativerai (Tamil)
Chandrashoor, asalu, halim (Hindi)
Garden cress seeds (English)
Halim shak, chandrashoor (Bengali)

Ambadi

Gongura (Telugu)
Pitwaa, ambad bhaji (Hindi)
Pulichakeerai (Tamil)
Pundi palle, pandi (Kannada)
Roselle leaves (English)
Taka bhendi, khata palanga (Odiya)

---

*These names might popularly refer to garden cress leaves.

Appendix

Kokum

Amsool, aamsul, ratamba, birund (Marathi)
Chinta (Telugu)
Mahada (Bengali)
Murugal (Tamil)
Punampuli, kodampuli (Malayalam)
Punarpuli, muragalu (Kannada)
Thekera (Assamese)
Tintali (Odiya)

A Note on the Author

Rujuta Diwekar is one of India's top nutritionists and the author of three bestselling books, including *Don't Lose Your Mind, Lose Your Weight*, the country's highest-selling diet book.

A Note on the Author

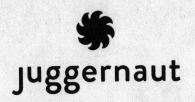

juggernaut

THE APP FOR INDIAN READERS

Fresh, original books tailored for mobile and for India. Starting at ₹10.

juggernaut.in

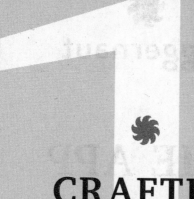

CRAFTED
FOR MOBILE
READING

*Thought you would never read a book
on mobile? Let us prove you wrong.*

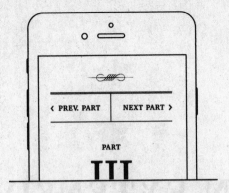

Beautiful Typography

The quality of print transferred
to your mobile. Forget ugly PDFs.

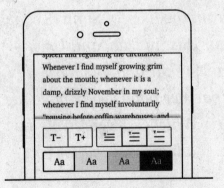

Customizable Reading

Read in the font size, spacing
and background of your liking.

AN EXTENSIVE LIBRARY

Including fresh, new, original Juggernaut books from the likes of Sunny Leone, Praveen Swami, Husain Haqqani, Umera Ahmed, Rujuta Diwekar and lots more. Plus, books from partner publishers and loads of free classics. Whichever genre you like, there's a book waiting for you.

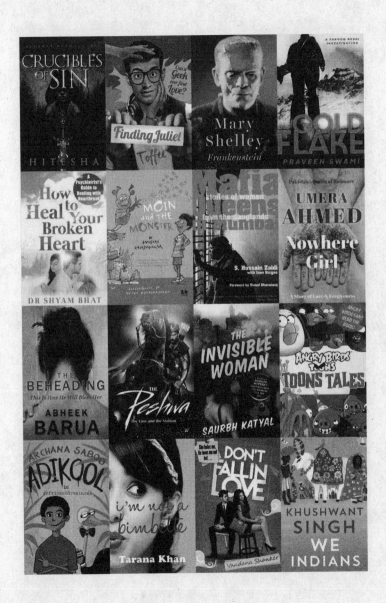

3

DON'T JUST READ; INTERACT

Thought you would never read a book on mobile? Let us prove you wrong.

Ask authors questions

Get all your answers from the horse's mouth.
Juggernaut authors actually reply to every
question they can.

Rate and review

Let everyone know of your favourite reads or
critique the finer points of a book – you will be
heard in a community of like-minded readers.

Gift books to friends

For a book-lover, there's no nicer gift than
a book personally picked. You can even
do it anonymously if you like.

Enjoy new book formats

Discover serials released in parts over
time, picture books including comics,
and story-bundles at discounted rates.
And coming soon, audiobooks.

4

LOWEST PRICES & ONE-TAP BUYING

Books start at ₹10 with regular discounts and free previews.

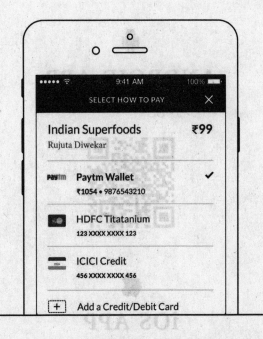

Paytm Wallet and Cards

Just connect your Paytm Wallet (or create one)
once and buy any book with one tap. Or pay
with your debit or credit card.

Click the QR Code with a QR scanner app
or type this link into the Internet browser
on your phone to download the app.

ANDROID APP

bit.ly/juggernautandroid

iOS APP

bit.ly/juggernautios

For our complete catalogue, visit www.juggernaut.in
To submit your book, send a synopsis and two
sample chapters to books@juggernaut.in
For all other queries, write to contact@juggernaut.in